HOW TO DRESS FOR MEN

The Modern Gentleman's Handbook to Mastering Stylish Living

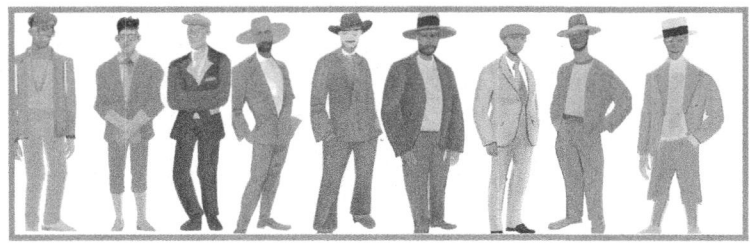

Madison Styles

Copyright © Madison Styles, 2023. All rights reserved.

This publication and its contents are protected by copyright laws and international treaties. No part of this publication may be reproduced or transmitted in any form or by any means, electronic or mechanical, including photocopying, recording or any information storage and retrieval system, without prior permission in writing from the copyright holder.

TABLE OF CONTENTS

Introduction: Style Has Power..................12
   The Benefits of Looking Good: Confidence, Success, and First Impression..................13
   The Essence of Men's Style Revealed: From the Foundation to Beyond..................17

Part I: Laying the Foundations..................21

Chapter 1: The Art of Dressing Classy..................22
   1.1 The Grace of Classic Clothing..................23
   1.2 Adopting Sartorial Customs..................24
   1.3 Crucial Pieces for a Classy Wardrobe..................26

Chapter 2: Mastering Professional Style..................29
   2.1 How to Dress for Success in the Corporate World..................30
   2.2 Business Casual: Getting the Balance Right....34
   2.3 Elevating Your Professional Look with the Power of Tailoring..................37

Chapter 3: Exuding Expensive Elegance..................41
   3.1 The Language of Luxury: Understanding Premium Materials..................42
   3.2 Accessorizing with Finesse: The Art of Subtle Opulence..................44
   3.3 Curating a High-End Wardrobe on a Budget....48

Chapter 4: Effortlessly Sexy: Unleashing Masculine Charm..................53
   4.1 The Charms of Confidence: Dressing to Attract...54
   4.2 The Art of Subtle Seduction: A Glimpse of Skin...58

4.3 Captivating Through Fitness: Sportsmanship with Flair.. 62

Part II: Beyond Borders: Cross-Cultural Dressing .. 66

Chapter 5: Celebrating Cultural Identity.................. 67

    5.1 Honoring Traditions: Dressing with Cultural Pride 68

    5.2 Navigating the World of Cross-Cultural Fashion... 73

Chapter 6: Seasons of Style: Dressing for Time and Climate..78

    6.1 Awakening in Spring: Easy Elegance for Blooming Days..79

    6.2 Summer Sophistication: Looking Hot while Remaining Cool.. 83

    6.3 Autumn Allure: Stunning Fall Fashion.............. 87

    6.4 Winter Man: Cozy Clothing for Cool Days........ 91

Part III: Dressing for Every Occasion........................ 96

Chapter 7: Casual Guy: Elevating Your Everyday Attire.. 97

    7.1 Effortless Cool: Navigating Casual Dress Codes. 98

    7.2 Dressing Down with Style: Beyond Denim and Tees.. 102

Chapter 8: The Art of Evening Glamour................. 107

    8.1 Black Tie Brilliance: Navigating Formal Dress Codes... 108

    8.2 Cocktail Connoisseur: Striking the Perfect Balance.. 111

Chapter 9: Groom and Groomsmen: The Perfect Wedding Ensemble...115

    9.1 Dapper Grooming: Dressing for Your Big Day 116

9.2 The Groomsmen's Handbook: Coordinated Looks for a Memorable Event.............................. 118

Chapter 10: Activewear Beyond the Gym: Athletic Excellence.. 122

10.1 Sporty Fashion: Dressing for Comfort and Performance......... 122

10.2 Athleisure Aesthetics: Combining Sophistication with Sport... 125

Part IV: Crafting Confidence Through Style........... 128

Chapter 11: The Confidence Code: Dressing for Self-Assurance...................................... 129

11.1 Unlocking Self-Esteem Through Your Wardrobe 130

11.2 How to Dress Confidently in Today's World.. 131

Chapter 12: Fit and Fabulous: Dressing for Different Body Types.. 134

12.1 Finding Your Perfect Fit: Celebrating Diversity... 135

12.2 Tailoring Advice: How to Dress for Your Individual Body.. 138

Chapter 13: The Power of Accessories: Upgrading Every Look.. 142

13.1 Getting the Hang of Men's Accessories: Watches and Wallets.. 143

13.2 The Magic of Ties, Pocket Squares, and More: The Subtle Impact................................145

Chapter 14: Fragrance and Beyond A Scent of Distinction.. 148

14.1 Men's Fragrance: The Art of a Signature Scent. 149

14.2 Deodorants, colognes, and Grooming Routines:

The Essentials.. 151

14.3 Choosing and Using Body Sprays, Deodorants, and Fragrances for Various Situations...................153

Chapter 15: Trendspotting: Including Contemporary Fashion in Your Wardrobe... 156

15.1 Interpreting Runway Trends: Adding High Fashion to Everyday Outfits.....................................157

15.2 Vintage Vibes: Reviving Timeless Pieces in Contemporary Ways... 161

Chapter 16: Style Evolution: Adapting to Changing Trends...166

16.1 Adopting Fashion's Fluidity: Dressing for the Future... 167

16.2 A Journey of Style Adaptation: Balancing Trends and Timelessness......................................169

Conclusion: Embrace Your Dapper Destiny........... 172

Enhance Your Everyday with Elegance: A Reminder to Keep Traveling in Style....................................... 174

Epilogue: Your Personal Style Manifesto..............178

Prologue: The Transformation of Carlton

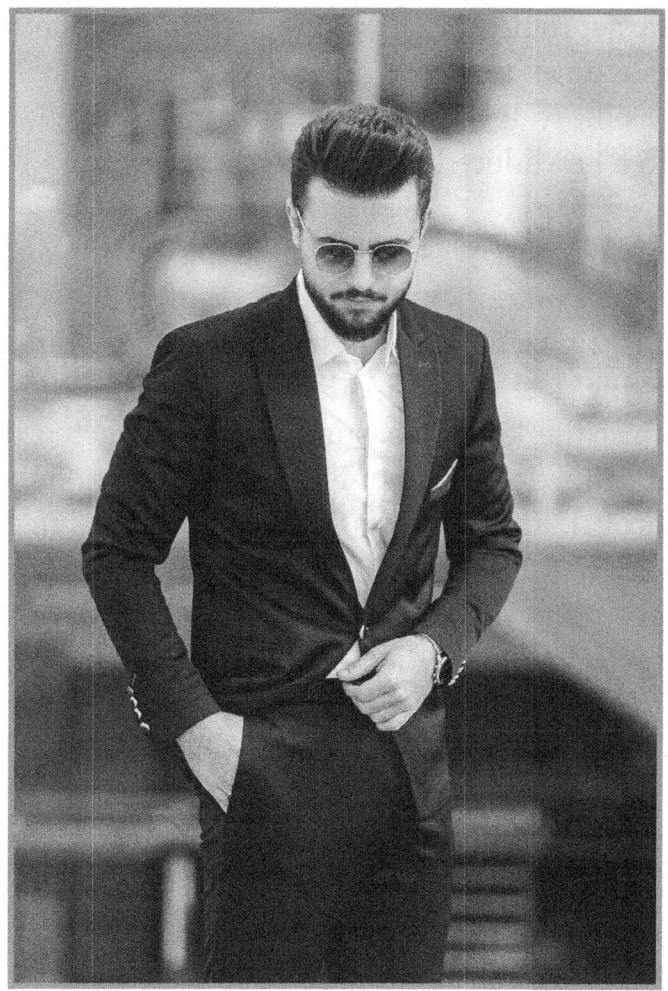

Although Carlton was a man of ambition, drive, and charisma, he encountered an unanticipated hurdle that caused his confident exterior to falter. Despite his successes, he was still faced with a problem that seemed to undermine his self-assurance. He pondered the riddle of dressing well as he stood in front of his closet with a bewildered look on his face.

Each morning was a challenge for Carlton as he had to contend with a variety of outfits that didn't fit well, mismatched accessories, and a nagging feeling of inadequacy. He desired to project the kind of assurance that attracted the admiring looks of his peers, the nods of approval from colleagues, and the sincere smiles of the ladies he met. He couldn't help but believe that his appearance didn't live up to his potential as he studied his mirror.

Then something changed. This book was given to Carlton by a friend; it was a ray of hope that would help him understand the complexities of men's clothing and alter his sense of style. Carlton read over its pages with skepticism but determination. What he discovered there was nothing short of a revelation—a thorough manual that dismantled the obstacles preventing him from being his best self in front of the world.

A surprising development started to take shape as Carlton immersed himself in the information in front of him. A route to dressing with purpose, finesse, and a fresh sense of identity was revealed by the book's ideas, which removed the layers of ambiguity. Carlton's confidence grew with each piece of advice he learned and each technique he perfected.

The days of rummaging through his closet and worrying over outfits that didn't embody him were long gone. Instead, Carlton started to create outfits that complemented his personality, goals, and desired image. He was awestruck by the effect of well-fitting clothing, the appeal of stylish accessories, and the subtle magic of color harmony. His shift from unsure to sophisticated was obvious; it went beyond his outward appearance and emanated from his whole being.

From friends who praised his increased sense of style to coworkers who treated him with newfound respect, the compliments came easily. Most significantly, Carlton observed a change in the way women interacted with him. They were drawn to him by his unmistakable presence and captivating appeal, which allowed them to connect in ways that were more natural and effortless than before.

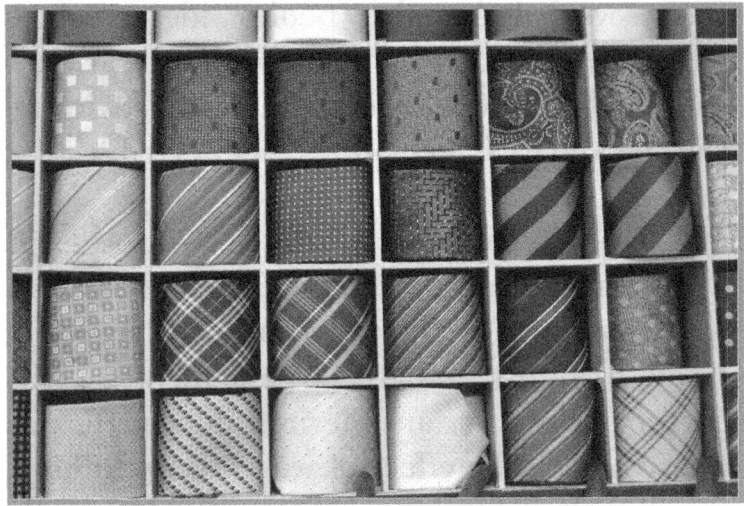

Imagine yourself in Carlton's position as you travel through the pages of "Dapper Decoded: The Ultimate Guide to Men's Dressing Mastery." Feel the development, accept the change, and be on the cusp of a style revolution that aims to boost your self-awareness, redefine your beauty, and give you the freedom to travel the world with a fresh sense of elegance.

You can learn how to dress like a man by using the advice in this book. You will learn how to dress with purpose, just like Carlton did, whether your goal is to captivate with your style, navigate new cultures, or exude timeless elegance. You are not alone as you set out on your life-changing adventure; Carlton's experience will serve as your road map and the knowledge contained in these pages as your lighthouse. Let's start this amazing journey together and open the door to a world where style is not just a reflection of who you are but also a potent declaration of your unwavering charm and confidence.

Introduction: Style Has Power

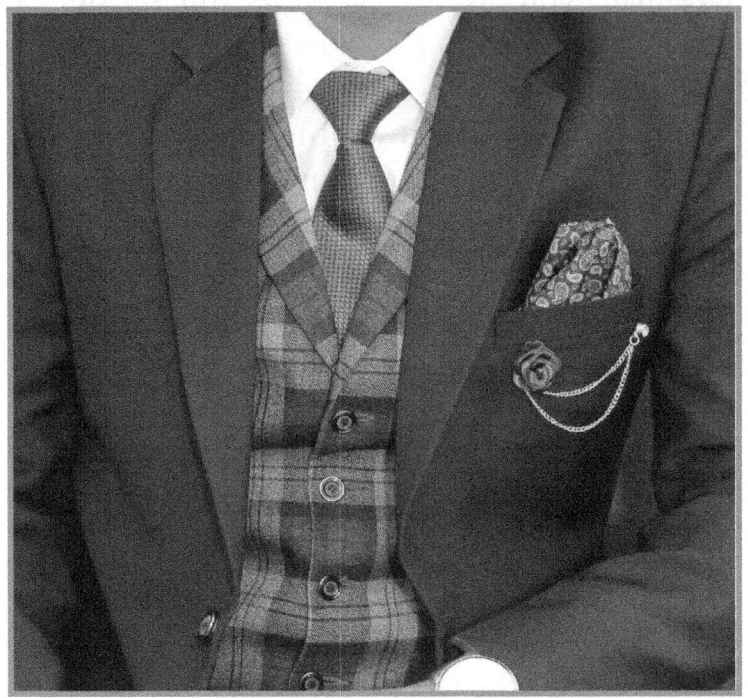

In a world where first impressions are frequently brief but significant, a man's choice of clothing has a tremendous impact that goes well beyond the obvious. When it comes to influencing views, boosting self-confidence, and opening doors to undiscovered chances, the power of style is a force to be reckoned with. This introduction reveals a tapestry woven with strands of self-assurance, achievement, and the possibility of transformation through peeling back the layers of the art of clothing.

The Benefits of Looking Good: Confidence, Success, and First Impression

Imagine a situation where people are gathering in a crowded space for a networking event. There are two intelligent, gifted, and accomplished men among them. However, the way they are dressed causes a stir in the crowd and elicits wildly divergent responses from individuals they come across.

The first man enters with a confident demeanor, his expertly made suit giving him a look of refinement and power. His demeanor speaks volumes, and his clothing serves as a reflection of his unflinching confidence. His aura exudes an unmistakable charisma that draws people to him, causing conversations to naturally drift toward him and partnerships to form without effort. He is the epitome of impeccable attire, and his presence radiates a magnetic power that commands respect.

The second man, who is similarly accomplished, tries to fit in with the crowd on the other side of the room. His outfit was untidy and his clothes didn't fit well, which diminished his potential. As he makes his way through the sea of interactions, conversations stall, relationships are transient, and his self-esteem suffers. The contrast between these two guys serves as a sobering reminder of the influence that grooming oneself well can have. This influence can either catapult one person to greatness or leave another trapped in a cycle of lost opportunities.

Taking pride in one's appearance demonstrates one's respect for themselves and their own abilities. It is a nonverbal declaration of one's identity, a call to attention from the outside world, and an affirmation of one's competence. The self-assurance that comes with looking well permeates all aspects of life, resulting in successful relationships, career advancements, and personal accomplishments. It is a language that communicates with the entire globe and amplifies one's voice without using any words.

The benefits of wearing properly go beyond personal empowerment and include the area of first impressions. According to research, first impressions are frequently made within milliseconds of meeting someone and are significantly impacted by appearance. So a man's choice of clothing serves as his shield, means of expression, and vehicle for presenting authenticity. The skill of wearing properly goes beyond mere aesthetics; it creates enduring impressions that can resonate for years to come by reshaping perceptions, igniting connections, and solidifying them.

The Essence of Men's Style Revealed: From the Foundation to Beyond

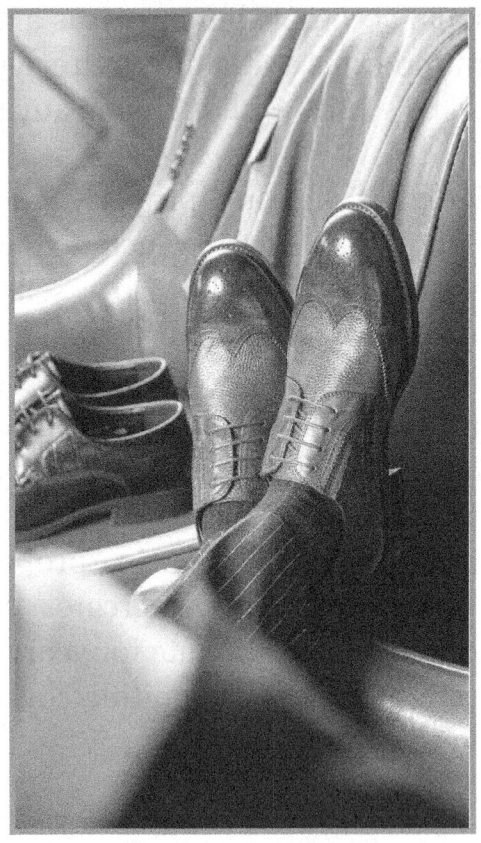

Men's fashion is a mesmerizing blend of creativity, purpose, and self-expression. This trip goes beyond simple aesthetics, eschewing fads, and frivolity in order to get to the very heart of a man's individuality. Style is a canvas on which a man paints his unique narrative, a narrative that expresses his values, ambitions, and aspirations to the world. Style is not only about dressing in the newest fashion trends or following social standards.

The foundation of men's style is the mastery of the essentials, which serve as the foundation for all outstanding ensembles. These fundamental components lay the platform for a wardrobe that shows personality and style, from choosing well-fitting clothes that enhance the body's silhouette to mastering the art of color coordination and accessorizing.

But men's fashion appeal goes well beyond the fundamentals. It explores the finer points of tailoring, the subtleties of fabric choice, and the skill of putting outfits together to produce styles that are both chic and adaptable. It explores the topic of cultural sensitivity, looking at how fashion can unite people and respect heritage while embracing modern trends. Whether it's controlling a boardroom, enthralling an audience, or leaving a lasting impression at a social gathering, it opens the door to dressing for success.

As we go through "Dapper Decoded: The Ultimate Guide to Men's Dressing Mastery," keep in mind that the essence of men's style is a dynamic dance between tradition and innovation, between timeless elegance and the modern aesthetic. Authenticity, personality, and charm are woven into a tapestry that creates a symphony of self-expression that resonates with both the wearer and those who are fortunate enough to come into contact with him.

So, set out on this explorational journey with an open mind and a curious heart. If some of the methods for dressing as a man described in this book do not sit well with you, you are free to disregard them and stick to the methods that do. Let the information in these pages help you navigate the nuances of men's fashion so you can harness the power of dressing well with assurance, refinement, and unwavering self-assurance. Let's take a journey together through a world where clothing becomes a tool of transformation, a monument to the amazing potential that exists within you, starting with the significance of that first impression and ending with the creativity that supports men's style.

Part I: Laying the Foundations

Chapter 1: The Art of Dressing Classy

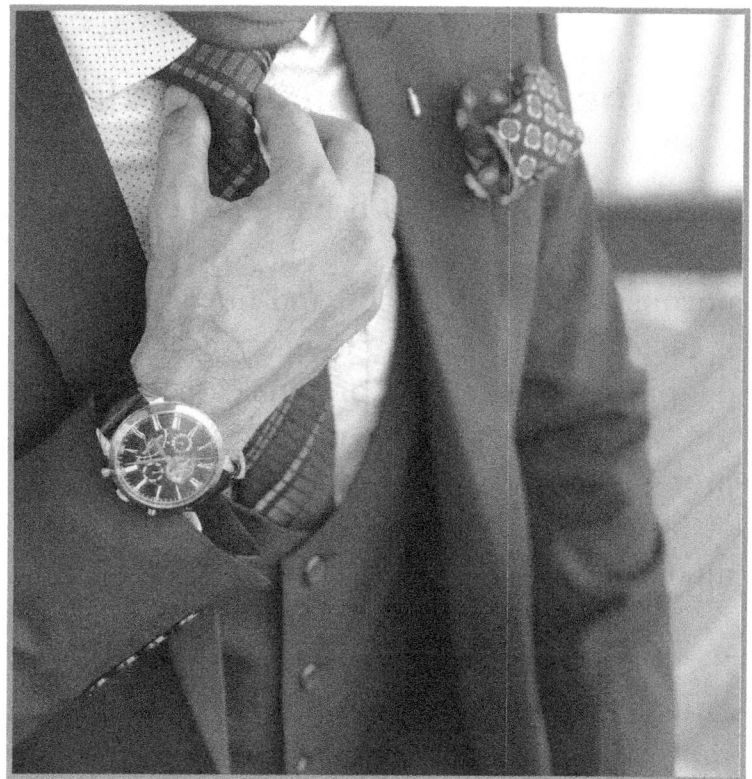

A timeless quality, elegance transcends fads and passing trends. It is a type of art that conveys profundity through subtle refinement and evokes a timeless sense of sophistication. This chapter delves into the complex fabric of classy clothing, examining the components that make it appealing and outlining the fundamental ideas that underpin this time-honored style.

1.1 The Grace of Classic Clothing

Dressing elegantly is a tribute to the appeal of timeless fashion, a world where style is unconstrained by the ebb and flow of fads and is instead anchored in a timeless aesthetic. The defining characteristic of timeless elegance is the ability to subtly combine the past and present to produce outfits that are reminiscent of bygone eras while still being relevant in the modern world.

By honoring the sartorial tradition that has influenced men's fashion over the years, a man can become the custodian of his own legacy by adopting timeless fashion. From the sartorial refinement of Old Hollywood to the ongoing influence of great personalities who have left an indelible stamp on the world of fashion, the fascination with well-fitted suits, pristine white shirts, and sophisticated footwear echoes across history.

1.2 Adopting Sartorial Customs

An appreciation for sartorial customs that have withstood the test of time is the cornerstone of sophisticated attire. The expertly cut suit, the artistically knotted tie, and the immaculately shined shoes are more than just articles of clothing; they are representations of a culture that values excellence, craftsmanship, and attention to detail.

Respect for the finer aspects of dressing, such as the way a pocket square is carefully folded, the choice of a correctly shaped lapel, and the significance of a strategically placed tie clip, is required to embrace sartorial traditions. It is a sort of art that elevates clothes above the every day and turns it into a precise symphony in which each component harmoniously contributes to the creation of a sophisticated outfit.

1.3 Crucial Pieces for a Classy Wardrobe

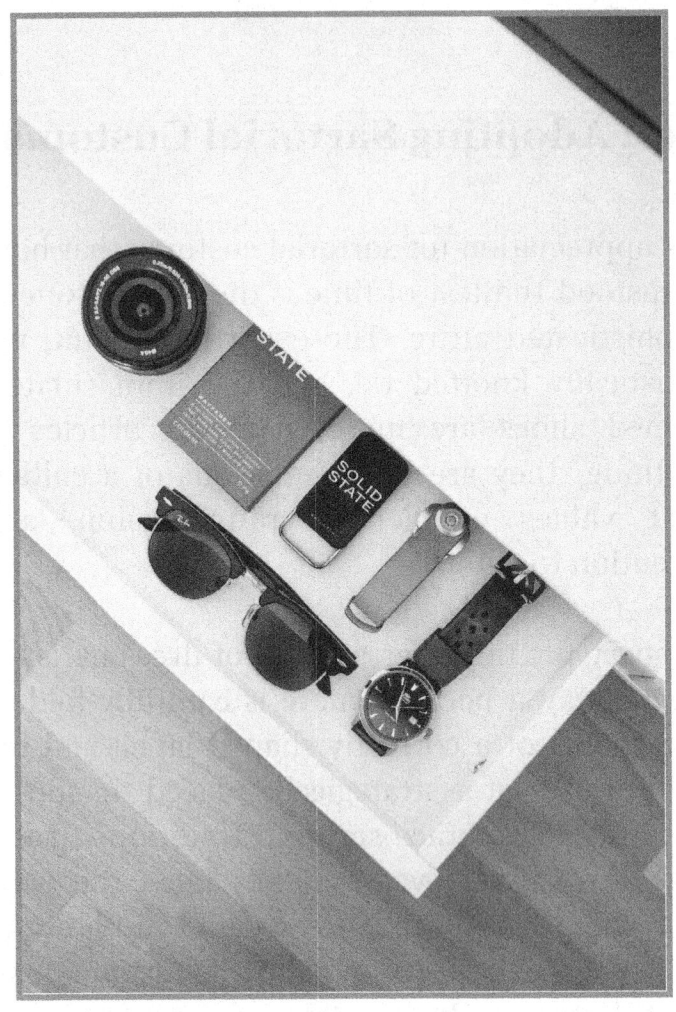

A selection of wardrobe staples that serve as the foundation of exquisite clothes are at the heart of wearing classily. These items can be worn for a variety of occasions and settings; rather, they serve as the foundation for an elegant and versatile wardrobe.

The classic suit, which embodies style and sophistication, is one of these necessities. A well-fitted suit conveys assurance and authority, making a statement that combines classic elegance with modern chic. Dress shirts made of high-quality materials go well with suits because their subtle patterns and textures give outfits depth and perspective.

To achieve stylish dress, footwear—often referred to as the cornerstone of an outfit—is essential. A pair of expertly constructed leather shoes boosts the entire appearance and highlights a man's attention to detail and dedication to a complete style. A man can add a touch of personal flair to his outfit with the help of accessories like ties, pocket squares, and cufflinks.

Keep in mind that the art of dressing classily is more than the sum of its parts as we draw to a close. It is a way of thinking that imbues every decision with intention and every combination with meaning. It is evidence that elegance is not a mystical idea reserved for a select few but rather a timeless journey that any man can take, each step leading him closer to a world where style is synonymous with grace, sophistication, and the everlasting charm of the well-dressed gentleman.

Chapter 2: Mastering Professional Style

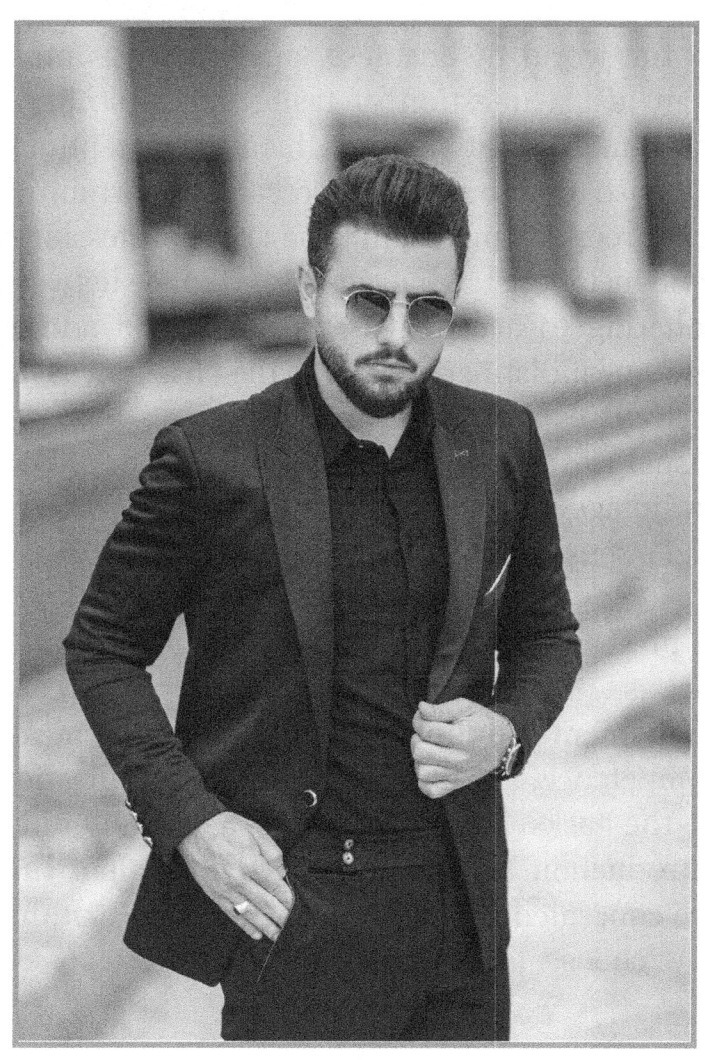

2.1 How to Dress for Success in the Corporate World

In the world of business, appearance is more than just a question of taste; it is a strategic instrument that may influence perceptions, increase credibility, and create opportunities for career advancement. The art of professional style includes striking a careful balance between adhering to accepted conventions and adding one's own distinctive flair to the ensemble. This section explores the subtleties of business casual wearing and offers tips on how to project an image that commands respect, authority, and a sense of purpose.

A professional's personal presentation should be as precise as a symphony, with each component working together to communicate competence, attention to detail, and dedication to the tasks at hand. It acts as a subliminal introduction to the knowledge and talent that are concealed beneath the surface. The clothing you choose for a professional setting conveys the message, "I am ready, capable, and poised to excel."

A thorough awareness of the company culture and the industry one operates is essential to mastering professional style. Expectations for suitable clothes may vary between industries and organizations. While some sectors choose a classic and formal style, others like a more laid-back but elegant look. It is crucial to research and adjust to these expectations because doing so shows a commitment to support workplace values and practices.

An impeccable suit is a necessary component of business style for the corporate gentleman. The suit serves as a canvas for conveying professionalism, so it is a perfect fit, and high-quality materials are essential. When choosing a suit, take into account the color, fabric, and style that are appropriate for your profession and your brand. While pinstripes or minor patterns can lend a splash of flair without sacrificing professionalism, navy and charcoal are adaptable options that show power.

Another essential element is the shirt, which needs to be crisp, well-ironed, and perfectly tailored. Choose traditional hues like white or light blue, and place an emphasis on quality over quantity. The tie serves as the centerpiece, allowing for a subtly stylish addition. Make a precise knot, making sure it matches the size of the lapel on your suit.

The finishing touch for a business outfit is frequently footwear, and leather dress shoes are the norm. Select a classy pair that matches the color of your suit and upholds the uniform style. Your attention to detail and dedication to professionalism is demonstrated by the condition of your shoes.

It's important to keep in mind that professional style encompasses more than just apparel as we negotiate the complex landscape of the corporate world. The importance of grooming and hygiene cannot be overstated, and a well-kept look shows commitment to personal excellence. Maintain a professional hairdo, trim your facial hair, and keep your nails clean and well-groomed.

Never forget that developing professional style involves mixing tradition with innovation, keeping to standards while integrating your own personality. It does not involve dressing in a rigid uniform. It involves making decisions that convey competence, assurance, and a firm commitment to the tasks at hand. Dressing for success in the workplace is more than just a fashion statement; it's a sign of professionalism, an admission that you're ready for any challenge, and a demonstration of your commitment to succeeding in business.

2.2 Business Casual: Getting the Balance Right

The distinction between formal and casual clothes is no longer as clear-cut in today's professional environment, giving rise to the idea of business casual. How to strike the fine balance between casual comfort and a professional air is the particular challenge presented by this sophisticated dress code. In this part, we explore the nuances of business casual wear and provide advice on how to maneuver through this flexible sartorial space while still projecting an air of sophistication.

Modern business professionals can embrace comfort without sacrificing a polished presentation thanks to business casual clothes. There are general principles that act as guiding principles amid the sea of possibilities, even though the rules may differ from one workplace to another. The goal is to appear polished and composed while maintaining a friendly personality that encourages teamwork and innovation.

The art of layering is the basis of business casual. Start with a well-fitted dress shirt and select colors that show your individual flair while also fitting in with the professional environment. Patterns and textures, such as subdued stripes or a herringbone weave, give your outfit more depth and complexity.

In a business casual situation, the necktie is no longer required, giving you the freedom to try open-collar shirts. Should you decide to wear a tie, nevertheless, think about a thinner width and a less formal pattern to go with the casual ambiance.

Dress slacks are the ideal complement to your shirt; choose ones in neutral hues like khaki, gray, or navy. These bottoms allow you to transition easily from work to after-hours engagements since they strike the right balance between formality and comfort.

Business casual footwear is still formal but more laid back. Excellent options that strike the ideal blend between class and comfort are leather loafers or derby shoes. Shoes are frequently the center of attention, so make sure they are kept in good condition.

It's important to embrace layers if you want to master business casual. A well-fitted blazer or sport coat boosts your look and adds a touch of sophistication that goes nicely with your shirt and pants. The blazer is a versatile item that can be dressed up or down, so having one in your business casual wardrobe is crucial.

It's important to keep in mind that professionalism should always be the guiding principle as we explore the art of business casual. Maintaining good grooming includes keeping your face clean-shaven or maintaining well-groomed facial hair, and making sure your haircut conveys class.

By adopting business casual, you open yourself to a world of possibilities for expressing your individual style while maintaining professional standards. Understanding the subtleties of the dress code and the sector you work in is essential to striking the correct balance between comfort and refinement. Never forget that dressing professionally but comfortably is a celebration of your ability to maneuver the complex world of modern professionalism.

2.3 Elevating Your Professional Look with the Power of Tailoring

Few things in the world of men's fashion have the same transformational potential as the craft of tailoring. The key ingredient that transforms an outfit from average to spectacular is the expertise of tailoring. This section highlights how tailoring may boost your appearance and give your clothing a sophisticated air while revealing the deep influence it has on your professional style.

Tailoring is a craft that entails modifying clothing to match your particular form, enhancing your silhouette, and emphasizing your strengths. When perfectly made, the suit, a staple of business wear, feels like a second skin. It conforms to your physique, resulting in crisp lines and an authoritative, self-assured profile.

The properly fitted dress shirt is one of the pillars of business attire. A sleek yet comfortable shape complements your dimensions while minimizing extra fabric from detracting from your polished appearance. The fit of a shirt can make all the difference. Be mindful of the length of the sleeves, making sure they expose only a hint of cuff while your arms are at your sides.

Even though they are frequently ignored, pants have enormous potential with the right tailoring. In order to provide a hint of elegance, the length should just touch the tops of your shoes. A comfortable fit is achieved while keeping a streamlined silhouette by tailoring the waist and seat.

Another canvas for the craft of tailoring is the blazer or sport coat. Important factors that affect the overall appearance are shoulder breadth, sleeve length, and general fit. Blazers with a tailored fit give you a polished appearance that heightens your stature and exudes refinement.

Despite appearing to be impervious to modification, footwear can benefit from small changes. Your dress shoes can be made more wearable by adding rubber soles for comfort or cushioned insoles for support, helping you walk with confidence all day long.

Beyond physical fit, tailoring's potency rests in the psychological impression it makes. When you wear clothing that has been expertly fitted to your body, you radiate confidence from the inside out. You appear to be someone who has given attention to even the slightest aspects as you stand straighter, walk with more assurance, and stand taller.

Keep in mind that tailoring is an investment in your image and self-confidence as you navigate the business world. Find expert tailors who are knowledgeable about the subtleties of fit and proportion, and work with them to produce clothes that enhance your professional presence. The craft of tailoring is your ticket to sartorial brilliance, whether it's a suit, a shirt, or a jacket. It's a journey that turns clothing into an extension of who you are, oozing the refinement and mastery that characterize the modern businessman.

Chapter 3: Exuding Expensive Elegance

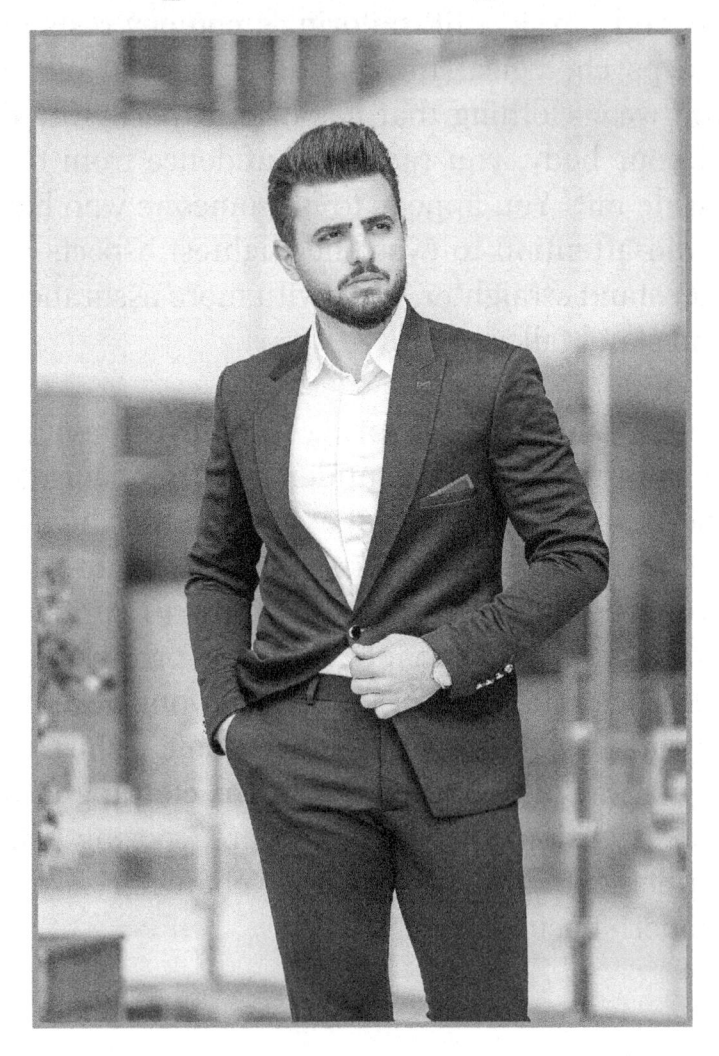

3.1 The Language of Luxury: Understanding Premium Materials

Beyond only the surface of clothing, the attraction of pricey elegance may be found in the very fabrics and textures that make up a garment. The body is draped in high-end fabrics that reflect the language of luxury, creating an opulent yet elegant tactile sensation. This chapter takes you on a tour through the world of luxurious fabrics and textiles, revealing the secrets of their making and highlighting how they can improve your sense of style.

It's similar to learning a new language to grasp luxury materials since they communicate intelligence, discernment, and an unconscious sense of quality. A keen eye, a passion for craftsmanship, and an uncompromising dedication to excellence are necessary for this language.

Silk, frequently referred to as the "queen of textiles," is a priceless substance that emanates sophistication and sensuality. Its silky feel caresses the skin and reflects light in an unmatched way. An outfit can become outstanding by adding a touch of luxury, such as a silk tie, pocket square, or dress shirt.

The fleece of the Kashmir goat is used to make cashmere, which is associated with luxury and comfort. A cashmere sweater or scarf, which is renowned for its softness and warmth, delivers an exquisite layer of opulence that envelops you in a cocoon of luxury, making every movement an expression of chic comfort.

When obtained from reliable sources and skillfully woven, wool is a durable material that is suitable for all seasons. Perfectly cut suits made of fine merino wool or virgin wool wrap the body with an unobtrusive delicacy, holding their shape and structure while radiating a timeless grace.

Exotic leathers provide accessories and footwear an air of distinction. Examples include beautiful calfskin or silky lambskin. A material that ages elegantly thanks to the rigorous tanning and treatment procedures develops a rich patina that conveys a message of enduring quality and sophistication.

It's crucial to recognize the minute details that set real premium materials apart from knockoffs when you set out on the adventure of oozing pricey elegance. Learn how to spot genuine luxury by becoming familiar with its distinguishing characteristics: smoothness, gloss, and attention to every stitch and finishing detail.

3.2 Accessorizing with Finesse: The Art of Subtle Opulence

A well-designed ensemble is punctuated with accessories, which give your overall appearance depth, personality, and a hint of grandeur. The art of accessorizing assumes an importance that goes well beyond aesthetics in the world of pricey elegance; it becomes a way to express uniqueness and give your outfit a feeling of refined sophistication.

The ability to enhance your look without overpowering it is the secret to accessorizing with grace. The goal is to compile a collection of accessories that go perfectly with your outfit, enhancing it without taking away from the composition as a whole.

Watches, frequently regarded as the pinnacle of male accessories, are more than just timepieces; they also serve as expressions of individual style and a sign of sophisticated taste. A well-selected watch may be a conversation starter and a statement piece that suggests your admiration for fine craftsmanship and attention to detail.

Despite their diminutive size, cufflinks have a big impact on the world of pricey elegance. These tiny pieces of artwork give you the chance to exhibit your uniqueness while elevating the look of your outfit. Choose styles that fit the occasion: understated elegance for formal occasions, and bolder, more expressive options for settings that value originality.

A tie bar, a seemingly unassuming item, adds a touch of refinement to your tie while also serving as a practical element. Although its primary function is to hold your tie in place, it also has an aesthetic influence, offering a refined touch that exudes fastidious attention to detail.

Finely created pocket squares made of silk or other high-end materials are an invitation to show your creativity. Precision folding and placement of a pocket square in your breast pocket add a splash of color and texture, giving your look personality and flair.

Premium leather shoes are highly regarded in the world of footwear. The footwear you choose can be a key component in elevating your complete appearance because it demonstrates your appreciation for quality and craftsmanship. Purchasing a quality pair of shoes—whether oxfords, derbies, or monk straps—is an investment in enduring elegance.

Keep in mind that the purpose of the art of accessorizing is intentionality, not excess. Each item should have a specific function, whether it be to improve the aesthetic appeal of your clothing, transmit a particular mood, or showcase your personality. The secret to subdued opulence is to create a sophisticated symphony that speaks to your sophisticated sensibilities by finding a balance that is harmonic among the components of your ensemble.

The mastery of fine fabrics and the dexterity of accessorizing become essential elements of your sartorial arsenal as you pursue pricey elegance. They are the threads that are used to create an image of discernment, refinement, and refined taste. This picture exudes a sophisticated aura that appeals to people who value the better things in life.

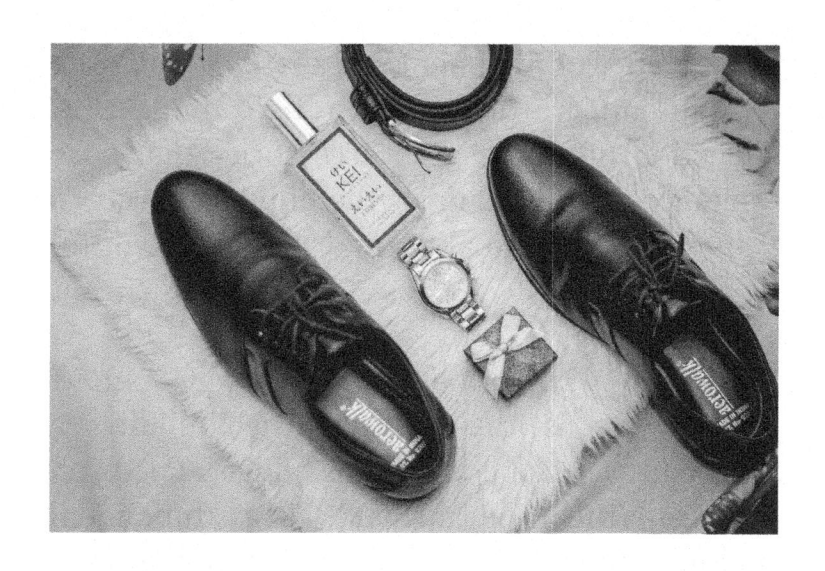

3.3 Curating a High-End Wardrobe on a Budget

Financial limitations do not always have to be an impediment to the appeal of an elite wardrobe. Curating a high-end wardrobe on a tight budget is not an impossible task; rather, it takes creativity, forethought, and a sharp eye for quality. In this section, we set out on a journey of research to learn how to build a chic and opulent wardrobe without going over budget.

The practice of judgment is essential to building a high-end wardrobe on a tight budget. A collection of clothes and accessories that ooze opulence is the result of the ability to discern value, prioritize quality, and make thoughtful decisions.

Strategic Investment: Making smart investments is the first step to building a high-end wardrobe on a tight budget. Focus on getting critical parts that act as functional building blocks rather than accumulating a large number of stuff. A classy wardrobe can be built around pieces like a well-tailored suit, a timeless white dress shirt, and a pair of fine leather shoes.

Vintage and Thrift: Vintage and thrift shops are troves of treasures just waiting to be found. Explore these areas with an open mind and look for classic artifacts that suit your own taste. The enduring quality that vintage ties, blazers, and leather accessories frequently display makes them valuable complements to your wardrobe.

Sales and Discounts: When navigating the world of sales and discounts, patience pays off. Pay close attention to end-of-season deals, clearance events, and seasonal promotions. With the help of these possibilities, you may upgrade your wardrobe without going over your spending limit by purchasing premium items for a small portion of what they originally cost.

When curating a high-end wardrobe on a tight budget, the adage "quality over quantity" becomes even more important. Choose a smaller number of well-made things that may be combined and matched to create a variety of looks. For example, a well-fitted blazer can easily move from formal situations to more informal ones, enhancing its adaptability.

Smart Accessorizing: Accessories have the ability to alter a look from ordinary to outstanding. Without spending money on a whole new outfit, you can add a sense of luxury to your wardrobe by strategically accessorizing. Your appearance can be enhanced and given an air of opulence with the use of a premium leather belt, an elegant tie, or a sleek pocket square.

Investigate do-it-yourself (DIY) crafts and customization to unleash your creativity. Adding distinctive buttons to simple dress shirts, personalizing pocket squares with embroidery, or refinishing leather accessories can give your wardrobe a sense of bespoke elegance that is exclusively yours.

Consignment shops and internet marketplaces provide a venue for purchasing previously used luxury products for a portion of their original price. These online stores give you access to a huge selection of high-end clothes and accessories that fit your posh fashion goals.

Alterations and Tailoring: The unsung hero of a high-end, reasonably priced wardrobe is tailoring. Even reasonably-cost clothing can be altered to create bespoke pieces that perfectly fit your body. Regardless of the original cost, tailoring guarantees that your clothing will appear and feel opulent.

Curating a high-end wardrobe on a tight budget demonstrates your ability to prioritize quality, make wise decisions, and express your own style through your clothing. Keep in mind that true luxury is not exclusively determined by cost; it also derives from respect for elegance, good craftsmanship, and self-assurance. By adhering to these guidelines, you can create an opulent-looking wardrobe without sacrificing your sense of financial restraint.

Chapter 4: Effortlessly Sexy: Unleashing Masculine Charm

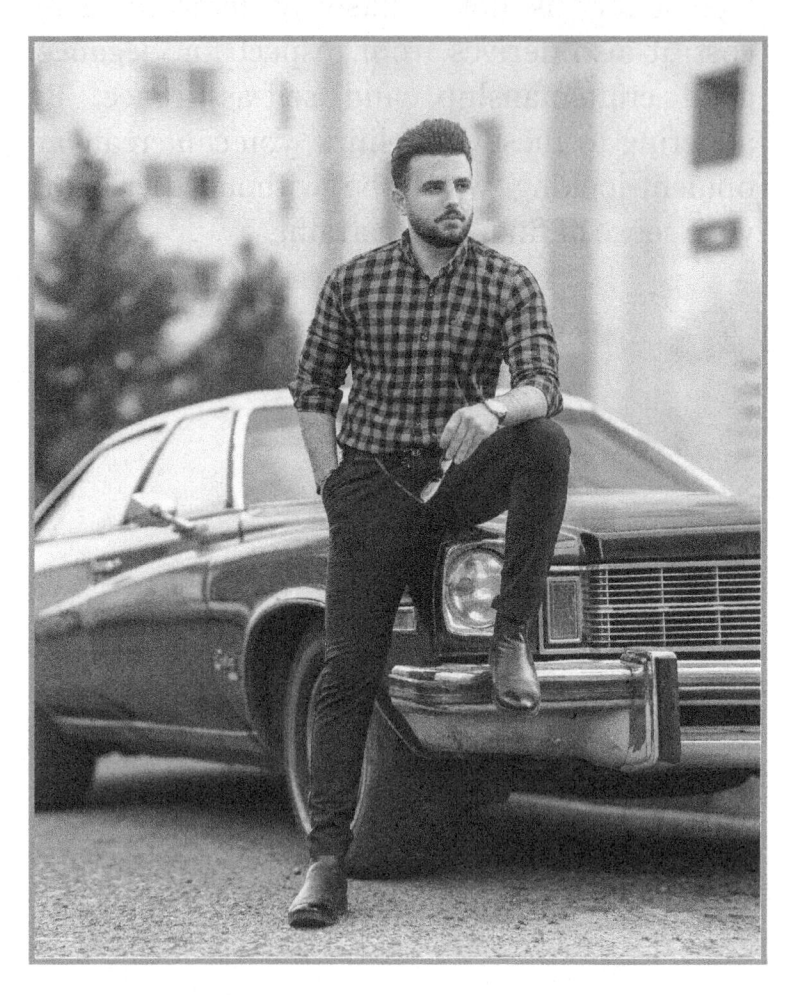

4.1 The Charms of Confidence: Dressing to Attract

The art of dressing becomes a potent instrument in radiating charm and igniting chemistry in the arena of attraction, where style extends beyond the mere aesthetic appeal of clothing. Wearing clothing that is effortlessly seductive involves more than just flashing flesh or dressing in a way that conforms to social standards of beauty; it also involves exuding confidence, embracing one's uniqueness, and creating an aura that attracts people to you. This section goes into the subtleties of dressing to attract and reveals how clothing and confidence work in harmony.

One characteristic stands out as the essence of effortless sexiness: confidence. Your self-assurance serves as the foundation for how you conduct yourself, connect with others and project energy. Embracing your individualism, appreciating your personality, and realizing that your unchanging sense of self-belief is the most enticing quality you can have are the first steps in the art of dressing to attract.

Dress to Fit Your Body: The key to an effortlessly attractive outfit is the way your clothes fit. The silhouette ought to highlight your advantages whilst yet feeling cozy. Whatever your physique—muscular, athletic, or lean—well-fitted clothing will highlight your proportions and highlight your body without being unnecessarily revealing.

The Power of Mystery: Leaving anything to the imagination can be very alluring. Choose clothing that hints at what is underneath without really showing it. Curiosity can be aroused and an air of interest can be created by a well-fitted shirt with the top button left casually undone, a sight of a well-toned forearm, or a faint suggestion of a tattoo.

Subtle Boldness: Details frequently reveal confidence. Subtle boldness shows that you aren't scared to embrace your personality, such as a special accessory or a splash of color in an otherwise understated outfit. These accents serve as conversation openers, enticing others to participate and learn more about the mysterious person in front of them.

Embrace Your Trademark: One of the most effective ways to achieve effortless sexiness is to identify and embrace your trademark style. Your signature style could be a certain brand of clothing, a particular color, or an individual approach to accessorizing. By becoming synonymous with your persona, this distinguishing characteristic makes you recognizable and alluring.

Attention to detail is the foundation of effortlessly sexy clothes, as are tailoring and grooming. Your clothing will fit you perfectly thanks to tailoring, enabling you to move with elegance and ease. An immaculate personal hygiene routine, well-maintained facial hair, and well-groomed appearance all contribute to your overall appeal.

The Importance of Comfort: Being at ease in your clothing contributes to genuine confidence. Pick textiles that are easy to move in and feel pleasant against your skin. People around you find it hard to resist your easy assurance when you are at ease.

Embrace Versatility: Effortlessly sensual clothing crosses stylistic barriers and adjusts to a variety of settings. Your wardrobe should be adaptable enough to handle many situations while still displaying your distinctive attractiveness, from casual outings to formal events.

Own Your Space: Effortless sexiness goes beyond appearance; it also refers to how you move around the environment. Maintain eye contact, stand tall, and show real interest in the people you are speaking with. You can convey confidence and appeal through your body language and manner.

Dressing to attract is about harnessing the power of confidence and self-assurance to create an enticing aura, not about complying with cultural expectations of sensuality. It's about realizing that the most alluring version of you is the one that exudes confidence and honesty. An extension of your inner charm, a declaration of your unapologetically unique identity, and an invitation for others to feel the magnetic energy you emanate are all made possible by effortlessly attractive clothing.

4.2 The Art of Subtle Seduction: A Glimpse of Skin

Men's fashion's subtle seduction technique goes beyond outright skin exposure; it entails purposeful flashes of skin that exude appeal and mystery. It's a delicate dance that calls for dexterity and an awareness of the influence of suggestion. A skillfully done exhibition of skin can arouse curiosity and leave a lasting impression on people who see you. The subtleties of this technique are revealed in this section, which also walks you through how to create subtle seduction while projecting an impression of sophistication.

The Collarbone Tease: The collarbone, a frequently disregarded erogenous region, serves as a backdrop for subtly seductive painting. Choose shirts with slightly broader necklines that expose the collarbone just a little bit. This subtle display of skin attracts attention without being overt, making it a seductive yet elegant option.

The Rolled Sleeve: The rolled sleeve is a quick and easy way to give your outfit a seductive touch. A hint of the forearm, which exudes a sense of power and masculinity, is visible when the sleeve is perfectly rolled up. This method works especially well with casual clothes since it gives your appearance a sense of unhurried confidence.

The versatility of the V-neck: When carefully chosen, the V-neck can be used as a weapon for subtly seducing people. An understated contrast that draws the eye downward is produced by layering a well-fitted V-neck shirt over a straightforward undershirt. This subtle reveal has more effect when it's coupled with a self-assured posture.

The Unbuttoned Shirt: This traditional gesture radiates a carefree, seductive air. A world of possibilities hidden beneath the cloth might be hinted at by leaving one or two buttons undone at the collar or chest. This strategy works best in social situations where a little lighthearted charm is suitable.

The Light Roll: When choosing jeans or trousers, take a light roll at the ankle into consideration. This understated aesthetic decision highlights your shoes while also showcasing a small portion of your ankle, which has an unexpected charm. This method works well in the summer because sleeves naturally catch the eye.

Layered Teasing: Using layers to add a hint of mystery can be effective. Over an undershirt, a semi-sheer shirt or an open-weave knit provides a seductive peek of flesh while preserving an impression of sophistication. This strategy gives your outfit more depth and texture, making it the perfect option for evening activities.

The Casual Blazer: A casual blazer blends effortlessness and sophistication when worn with a plain T-shirt. The jacket lends a touch of sophistication, and the T-shirt's exposed V-neck gives off an equally alluring impression of casual charm.

Men's style's creative restraint is what subtle seduction is all about; it's the thin line between showing and concealing, between suggestion and revelation. The secret is to preserve an air of mystery and let your clothing arouse interest and the imagination. By mastering the skill of subtly seducing a person, you may change your style into a compelling story that communicates a lot without saying anything.

4.3 Captivating Through Fitness: Sportsmanship with Flair

A dynamic aesthetic that emphasizes both form and function has emerged as a result of the confluence of athletic style and fashion. Utilizing athletic clothing's visual effect while adding flair outside of the gym is key to captivating people via fitness. It's about demonstrating your commitment to fitness while projecting a sense of style and confidence. This section guides you through the best methods to incorporate sports features into your regular outfits while delving into the subtleties of athletic style with flare.

enhanced Activewear: When enhanced with thoughtful fashion, activewear transcends the boundaries of the gym. Choose athletic clothing that fits well and enhances your figure. A sleek tracksuit or pair of joggers combined with a perfectly tailored hoodie makes for a casual, sporty, and unquestionably fashionable look.

Sneakers as a Fashion Statement: Sneakers have developed from basic sporting shoes to sought-after fashion accents. Choose sneakers that express your personality by having distinctive designs, striking colors, or unexpected embellishments. These footwear options contribute to your overall appearance while giving your outfit a hint of athleticism.

Sportswear that is layered: Sportswear that is layered over more formal attire gives the outfit a layered, dynamic appearance. Wearing a thin athletic jacket over a fitted shirt and pairing it with slim-fit trousers or chinos demonstrates how to successfully combine casual and formal aspects.

The modern marvel known as the athleisure suit blends the comfort of activewear with the beauty of a suit. Both formal and informal settings benefit from the relaxed sophistication that a well-fitted jacket and tailored sweatpants or joggers offer.

Purposefully accessorize: Accessorizing gives you the chance to add flair to your athletic look. Choose accessories that fit your energetic persona, such as slim sports watches, rubber or silicone bracelets, or light backpacks. These accents highlight your dedication to fitness while complementing your entire appearance.

Monochromatic Mastery: Ensembles in one color are an effective way to express a sense of cohesion and purpose. Build your ensemble around a single color scheme, adding athletic-inspired clothing and sporty accents like sneakers. This method produces a unified and visually arresting look.

Use technical textiles creatively: Technical fabrics, frequently connected with athletic apparel, have entered the mainstream of fashion. Comfort and style are both offered by clothing made of breathable or moisture-wicking materials. Add technical elements to your outfit for a hint of sporty sophistication.

Embracing your dedication to a healthy lifestyle and expressing it through your personal style is how to be captivating through fitness. It exudes confidence and vigor as a celebration of movement, athleticism, and self-improvement. You can build an outfit that not only demonstrates your commitment to fitness but also your skill in mastering the mix of style and athleticism by adding sports aspects and a touch of flair to your regular wear.

Part II: Beyond Borders: Cross-Cultural Dressing

Chapter 5: Celebrating Cultural Identity

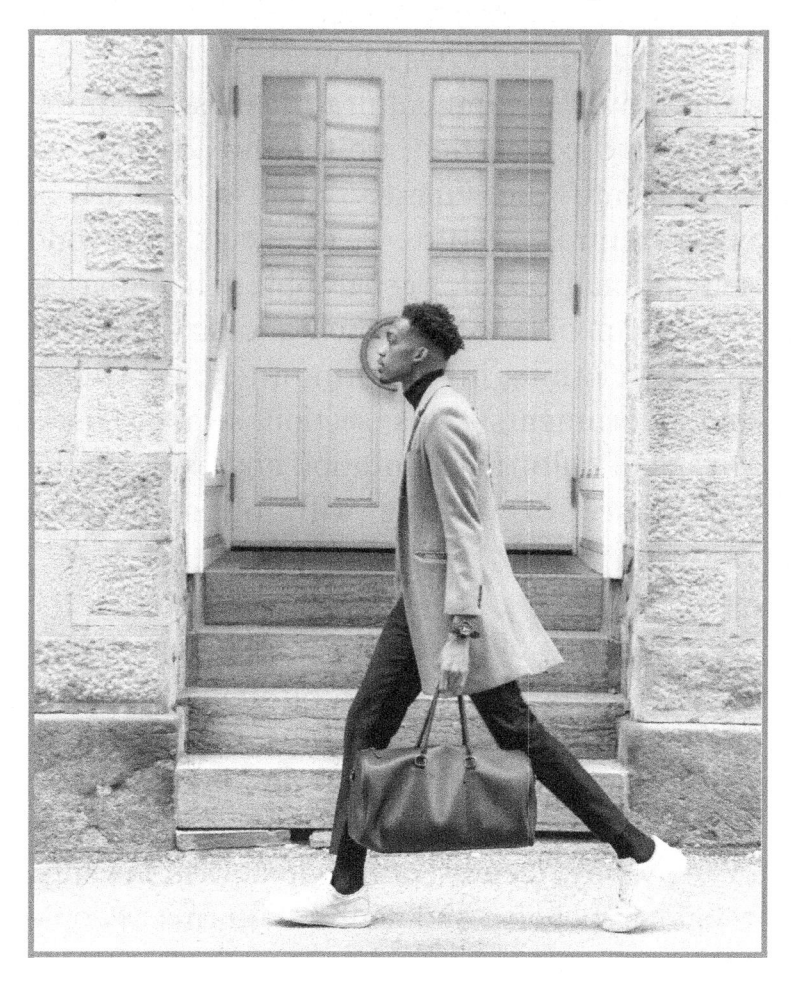

5.1 Honoring Traditions: Dressing with Cultural Pride

Dressing becomes a means of expressing one's ancestry, embracing cultural roots, and honoring ancestor traditions in a world that values diversity and cultural richness. Identity, pride, and connection are the threads that are woven into the tapestry that is the art of cross-cultural attire. It cuts beyond generational and geographic boundaries, enabling people to wear their ancestry as a part of their clothing in the form of textiles, colors, and adornments. This section sets off on a voyage of cultural exploration and explores the importance of wearing with pride in one's culture.

A Symphony of Symbols: A rich tapestry of symbols and motifs with profound meaning frequently weaves itself into the fabric of cultural identity. Traditional designs, elaborate embroideries, and native prints express stories visually by representing historical events, religious beliefs, and cultural norms. People that wear clothing with these symbols on it embody the legacy of their ancestors and carry a bit of their culture with them.

The Art of Fusion: Adhering flexibly to one tradition is not the only aspect of cross-cultural attire. A dynamic confluence of elements, it successfully combines innovation and tradition. Combining modern interpretations of traditional attire with modern components results in ensembles that honor cultural origins while embracing the fluidity of the present.

Redefining Identity: In the contemporary world, redefining identity involves dressing with cultural pride. By incorporating traditional aspects into everyday clothing, people make a statement about their identity that reads, "I am rooted in tradition, yet I am a product of my time." They also celebrate their lineage and push the limits of what is considered to be acceptable identification.

Dressing in traditional dress serves as a trigger for cultural revitalization. It rekindles interest in traditions that could be losing favor, preserves them, and passes the legacy on to younger generations. It serves as a link between the past and the present, fostering a sense of community and preserving cultural heritage.

The Language of Colors: Colors have a great deal of cultural meaning and are frequently used to express feelings, social standing, or spiritual beliefs. The color scheme of clothing serves as a visual representation of cultural identity. Subdued tones may represent melancholy and meditation, while vibrant hues highlight joy and festivity. People have a silent dialogue with their roots when they choose colors that are symbolic of their heritage.

Celebrating Festivals and Rituals: Festivals and rituals are powerful platforms for the expression of cultural identity. During these festivals, traditional clothing takes center stage, bringing communities together and reaffirming shared beliefs. When people dress with cultural pride for these holidays, it serves as a reminder of the continuing value of tradition in a dynamic environment.

Traditional clothing frequently displays exceptional craftsmanship and artistic talent. Textiles made by handweavers, elaborate beadwork, and painstaking needlework are examples of the talent and commitment of artists. When people wear these items, they not only respect their culture but also the skilled hands that created them.

A Generational Dialogue: Wearing clothing with cultural pride helps to close generational divides and promotes communication between the past and the present. Younger generations can engage in intergenerational discussions that deepen their understanding of their cultural inheritance and help them reconnect with their roots and heritage.

A Global Tapestry: Geographic barriers are not a barrier to cross-cultural attire. It weaves a fabric of common experiences, respect for one another, and understanding of different cultures. People from many origins add to a tapestry of human stories that highlight the beauty of our interconnected world as they appreciate their own heritage and learn about others.

Wearing clothing with cultural pride is a way to honor one's ancestors, celebrate one's individuality, and reflect the rich history of humanity. It's an opportunity to interact with others, go on a journey of self-discovery, and delve more into cultural variety. People who wear clothing reflective of their heritage become ambassadors of cultural diversity, carrying the stories of their ancestors and incorporating them into modern life.

5.2 Navigating the World of Cross-Cultural Fashion

The borders between cultures become permeable in a world that is becoming more connected, resulting in a lively panorama of cross-cultural fashion. A delicate dance of aesthetics, symbolism, and the deep influence of clothing as a means of communication is the art of merging cultures through clothes. It serves as a tribute to the beauty that results from the blending of various cultures, as well as a celebration of shared experiences and an exploration of uncharted territory. This chapter explores the complexities of navigating the realm of cross-cultural fashion and provides tips on how to politely and tastefully combine elements from many cultures.

Cultural Synthesis: Blending cultures through clothing is not just about copying styles verbatim; it's also about creating a synthesis that preserves the spirit of each culture while creating a unified whole. This strategy entails identifying resonances and commonalities between many traditions to facilitate their seamless fusion.

Cross-cultural clothing can be used to express stories in ways that go beyond language. Each piece of clothing becomes a chapter in a story that describes the wearer's journey, experiences, and appreciation for many cultures. Individuals build ensembles that express a complex sense of identity by carefully choosing and fusing elements from several cultures.

The Function of Accessories: Accessories are essential to cross-cultural fusion because they provide a way to incorporate elements from different cultures without overpowering the ensemble. The focal point that unites several ethnic influences can be a traditional accessory, such as a scarf, necklace, or headdress.

Prints, patterns, and textiles: These visual languages are used to communicate cultural history. Your clothing gains an eclectic feel when you incorporate textiles with distinctive motifs or weaving patterns from many cultures. The secret is to find a balance that brings out the distinctive qualities of each component while forming a unified whole.

Fusion of color palettes: Colors have cultural importance all around the world. Using a variety of colors in an outfit can showcase the richness of ethnic diversity. Bright colors placed next to one another can inspire a sense of unity and provide a visually stunning ensemble that honors several traditions.

Respecting Origins: It's crucial to respect each element's historical context and meaning when blending civilizations. Learn the meaning of various cultural components so that you can avoid unintended appropriation or misinterpretation. You show a sincere appreciation for the cultures you are combining by knowing the backstories of each element.

Building Bridges: Fashion that crosses cultural boundaries has the potential to foster respect and understanding. It's a means to interact with people from different backgrounds in a conversation that cuts beyond language boundaries. You encourage conversations that celebrate our shared humanity by dressing in a way that represents many cultures.

Cross-cultural fashion is an example of cross-cultural exchange that transcends national boundaries. It's a chance to have a constant dialogue with the rest of the world while exhibiting the beauty of other cultures and encouraging people to discover and value the depth of the human experience.

Fashion's ability to meld cultures allows for unmatched personal expression. It's an opportunity to put together an ensemble that expresses your uniqueness, ideals, and the external influences that have influenced your worldview. By embracing cross-cultural fusion, you develop a personal sense of style.

The celebration of cross-cultural dress highlights how interrelated all people are. It serves as a visual illustration of the beauty that results from the fusion of different civilizations, deepening our awareness of the world and our place in it. People can put together ensembles that stand as live examples of the world's diverse cultures by navigating the world of cross-cultural fashion with tact, respect, and a sincere desire to learn and connect.

Chapter 6: Seasons of Style: Dressing for Time and Climate

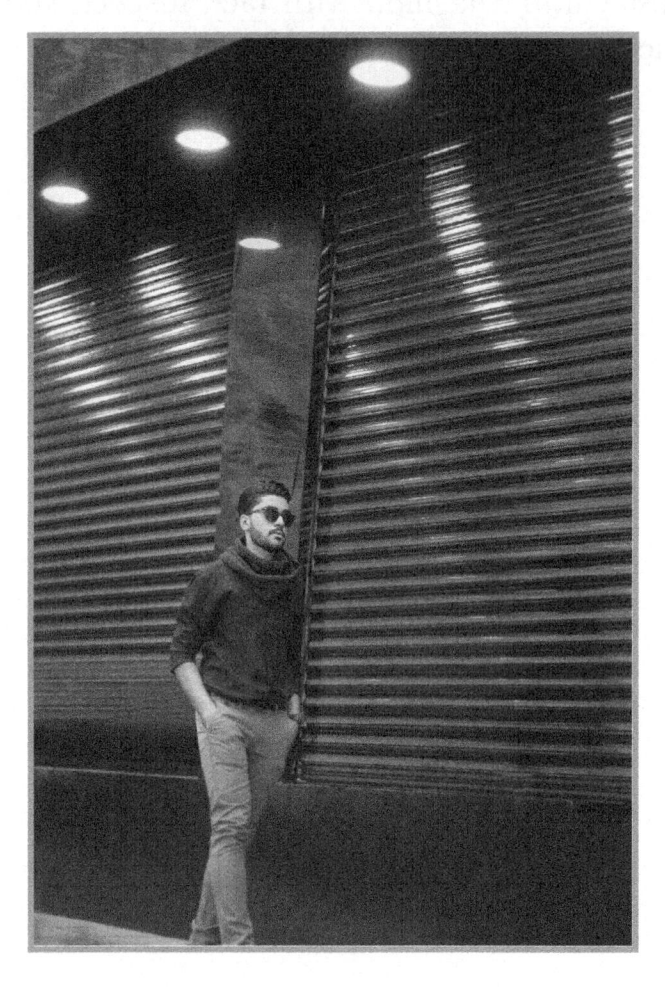

6.1 Awakening in Spring: Easy Elegance for Blooming Days

A rush of brilliant hues, budding flowers, and the prospect of warmer days are all signs of spring, a season of renewal and rejuvenation. Our approach to style changes along with how nature changes. This transformation is reflected in spring clothing, which is marked by a sense of lightness, fun, and an embrace of nature. This chapter explores the art of dressing with carefree elegance during the springtime and provides tips on how to capture the spirit of the blossoming days.

Embracing Floral Fantasies: Springtime is linked with blooms. You can embody the spirit of the season and create a visual representation of the planet reawakening by incorporating floral motifs into your clothing. Floral designs add a touch of nature's craftsmanship to your outfit with their range of bold and delicate blooms.

Spring is a canvas painted in delicate pastel colors, including mint green, blush pink, baby blue, and buttery yellow. Use these delicate hues to build an outfit that reflects the delicate beauty of spring. Shirts, pants, and accessories in pastel hues convey a feeling of tranquility and freshness.

Light Layers: The weather in spring can be erratic, varying from chilly mornings to warmer afternoons. The secret to easily adjusting to these changes is wearing light layers. To adapt to shifting temperatures, a thin cardigan, a sharp jacket, or a chic trench coat can be added or withdrawn with ease.

Dresses are the epitome of effortless spring grace. Choose gowns that embody the season, such as wrap dresses, A-line dresses, or flowing maxi dresses. Playful patterns and feminine accents, like lace or ruffles, give your outfit a whimsical and elegant feel.

The footwear of spring seeks a balance between fashion and utility. Accept casual footwear for men such as ankle boots, loafers, or canvas sneakers. With these options, you can experience the awakening world without sacrificing comfort.

The Versatile Scarf: A thin scarf may bring style and warmth to your outfit as a springtime accent. Choose scarves with jolly prints or delicate patterns to add a touch of beauty to your outfit. A scarf adds color and comfort to your attire when draped over your shoulders or loosely wrapped around your neck.

Flowing textiles: Spring asks for textiles that mimic the motion of the natural world. Select chiffon, silk, or light cotton fabrics that allow you to move gracefully and catch the mild wind. The essence of spring's unfolding beauty is embodied by flowing skirts, blouses, or wide-leg jeans.

Natural Accessories: The coming of spring encourages us to reconnect with nature, and accessories can help us do that. To give your outfit an organic feel, incorporate natural materials like woven belts, shell earrings, or wooden bangles.

The Benefits of Rainwear: Spring rains serve as a reminder of the power of nature to sustain life. You can welcome the rain while looking stylishly prepared if you have a chic umbrella, a water-resistant jacket, or waterproof shoes.

Dressing elegantly yet carelessly in the spring is a tribute to the wonder of change and renewal. It's an opportunity to celebrate the changing scenery and reflect the spirit of the rebirth of the season in your outfit. You can create outfits that perfectly embody the joy of spring's rebirth by including floral motifs, pastel colors, light layers, and flowing fabrics.

6.2 Summer Sophistication: Looking Hot while Remaining Cool

A style shift that strikes a balance between ease and manly elegance is called for by the summer, a season of sun-kissed days and pleasant evenings. The chance to demonstrate a particular style of sophistication that flourishes in the heat increases as the temperature rises. It takes skill to stay cool in the summertime while still radiating unmistakable attractiveness. The subtleties of summertime attire are discussed in this part, along with tips on how to balance fiery style with comfortable casual wear.

Lightweight Layers: Even though the summer sun can be very hot, the change from the outside heat to the air conditioning inside a building can cause a temperature difference. The solution to this sartorial conundrum is light layering. Choose breathable items like sheer cover-ups, linen jackets, or open-knit sweaters for a touch of warmth.

Use breathable textiles to keep cool in the heat and to keep your skin feeling comfortable. Seersucker, chambray, linen, and cotton are all wonderful options that provide a chic means of escaping the summer heat. These materials not only keep you cool but also give your outfit a carefree sophistication.

Summer dresses are the pinnacle of effortless grace. These outfits, which range from breezy shirt dresses to flowing maxi dresses, provide both comfort and style. Choose dresses with airy materials, wacky designs, and feminine silhouettes that reflect the season.

Cool and Crisp Whites: Summer sophistication is always embodied in crisp white apparel. Whether it's a lightweight blazer, a pair of white pants, or a cut white shirt, these items have a classic beauty about them. White serves as a blank canvas for accessories and encourages color experimentation.

Swimwear: Beach vacations and poolside relaxing are common summer activities. Stylish swimming trunks that radiate sophistication will up your swimwear game. Choose timeless one-pieces with elegant patterns to show off your sense of summer style.

Bold Accessories: Accessorizing is a great way to add refinement to your summer wardrobe. A simple suit may be made into a fashion statement with the help of dramatic sunglasses, big hats, and delicate jewelry. Select items that not only add style to your look but also offer useful sun protection.

Fashionable Footwear: Summertime footwear creates a mix between fashion and utility. Select footwear that matches your outfit, such as open-toe sandals, espadrilles, or loafers, and allows your feet to breathe. These options are adaptable complements to your summer wardrobe because they go from day to night with ease.

You should only use effortless makeup if you are at ease doing so. Summertime makeup should embrace a fresh, natural appearance. Choose lightweight makeup that doesn't feel heavy to complement your features, such as waterproof mascara and delicate lip tints. A glowing complexion that can survive the summer heat is the aim.

Embracing Vibrant Colors: The summer is a great time to try out bold designs and bright hues. By mixing hues like coral, turquoise, and brilliant yellow into your outfit, you can embrace the vivacious spirit of the season. Summer sophistication is captured in playful designs and vibrant colors.

Summer sophistication captures the essence of the season's carefree attitude while embracing a refined look. It is a seamless fusion of ease and elegance. You may put together outfits that perfectly capture the art of remaining cool while still appearing unbelievably hot by choosing breathable fabrics, adding classic swimwear, and embracing cool whites.

6.3 Autumn Allure: Stunning Fall Fashion

Autumn, a time of change and transition, brings with it a kaleidoscope of warm hues, crisp air, and an urge for contemplation. Our outfit changes as nature transforms, moving toward comfortable layers and a color scheme influenced by the changing leaves. The goal of autumn allure is to capture the attraction of the season, where clothing expresses ease, sophistication, and a connection to nature. This section explores the nuances of fall attire and offers advice on how to incorporate the beauty of autumn into your personal style.

The Warmth of Layering: Autumn is synonymous with layering, which enables you to gracefully adjust to rapidly changing temperatures. Use scarves to cover comfortable knit dresses or lightweight sweaters and fitted blazers to embrace the art of layering. Layering gives your outfit depth and keeps you at a comfortable temperature.

Rich & Earthy Tones: Rust, mustard, deep burgundy, and forest green make up the symphony of warm, earthy tones that make up the fall color pallet. To embody the spirit of the season, include these hues in your attire. These hues inspire a cozy feeling and work in perfect harmony with the shifting surroundings.

Cozy Knitwear: Fall is the ideal season to treat yourself to expensive knitwear. Pick warm, cozy items like turtlenecks, cable-knit cardigans, and thick sweaters. Knitwear gives your ensembles more depth and texture, giving them a tactile charm.

Elegant Outerwear: As the temperature drops, outerwear becomes more prominent. Invest in classic coats and jackets that will keep you warm and add style to your outfit. Outerwear creates a fashion statement, whether it's a timeless trench coat, a fitted pea coat, or a striking leather jacket.

Textured fabrics: Fall fashion benefits from textures that mimic the season's tactile feelings. Accept materials like tweed, suede, corduroy, and wool that give your clothing depth. These textures accentuate the richness of autumn while adding aesthetic interest.

Versatile Boots: The fall season is known for its chic footwear, and boots are the ideal option. Boots come in a range of heights from ankle to knee, adding comfort and flair to your fall wardrobe. To create a variety of looks, experiment with different styles and materials.

Statement Accessories: In fall fashion, accessories take center stage. Oversized scarves, bold belts, and chunky jewelry that adds personality and flair can elevate your look. These accessories are discussion starters and attract attention.

Plaids, houndstooth, and animal patterns are a few examples of prints that are inspired by autumn. These patterns give your clothing a retro feel and go well with the cozy ambiance of the season.

Embracing Layers in cosmetics: Many of the male celebs I am familiar with wear cosmetics before to any event, show, or other occasion. Some even continue to wear makeup on a regular basis. However, you shouldn't do this if you are not comfortable doing so, as comfort is an essential component of dressing like a man. Deeper, richer tones that reflect the changing leaves are embraced in fall makeup. Create an autumnal makeup look by experimenting with warm eyeshadows, berry-toned lipsticks, and a hint of bronzer.

Hairstyles for Transition: Fall hairstyles exude a carefree grace. Choose hairstyles with textured updos, sleek ponytails, or tousled waves to embody the season's laid-back feel while still looking chic.

Autumn allure is a celebration of the comforting nature of the season as well as its transforming beauty. Layering, rich colors, comfortable knits, and textured fabrics are all used to create looks that reflect the allure of fall. Autumn transforms into a canvas for expressing your style through the prism of nature's changing hues as you make your way from summer to winter.

6.4 Winter Man: Cozy Clothing for Cool Days

The earth is covered in snow during the winter, a time of magic and stillness, and it beckons us to enjoy the comforts of warmth and cozy. Fashion serves as a medium for communicating coziness, elegance, and a hint of grandeur as the temperatures decrease. The goal of winter wonderland fashion is to create warm, magical looks that radiate warmth. This section examines the art of dressing for the winter and offers advice on how to brave the chilly weather while still looking chic.

Luxurious Layering: The key to winter dressing is layering intelligently. Warmth-retaining undergarments should be worn first to keep heat near your body before adding comfy sweaters, turtlenecks, and cardigans. Finish with a chic coat or parka to keep you warm and show off your winter fashion skills.

Playful Prints and Patterns: Add some color and brightness to your winter wardrobe by wearing prints and patterns that are fun and playful. These patterns provide visual appeal and encapsulate the spirit of the season, whether it's a traditional Fair Isle sweater, a tartan scarf, or a houndstooth coat.

Rich Textures: The many luxurious textures that winter brings will make your clothing stand out. Accept luxurious and comfortable materials like velvet, cashmere, wool, and faux fur. These textures have a tactile appeal that captures the cozy atmosphere of the time of year.

Elegant Outerwear: Winter outerwear makes a fashion and practical statement. Choose a distinctive coat that not only enhances your look but also offers weather protection. Your winter wardrobe's focal point is a well-fitting wool coat, a cushioned puffer jacket, or a tailored pea coat.

Winter items are both functional and fashionable. Pick warming and fashionable accessories like knit scarves, gloves, and beanies to complete your look. Don't be scared to play around with various textures and colors.

Winter footwear that serves a purpose creates a mix between fashion and utility. Select insulated boots that go with your winter wardrobe and offer grip on icy surfaces. Your footwear, whether they are traditional leather boots or waterproof snow boots, should keep you warm and dry without sacrificing style.

Leggings and tights with layers: Layering also includes your lower body. For extra warmth, wear leggings or thermal tights with your dresses and skirts. You may continue to wear your favorite items while being warm by layering them.

Statement Scarves: A single flourish can completely change the way you look with this multipurpose winter accessory. Choose warm-weather accessories like giant blanket scarves, plush infinity scarves, or chic silk scarves.

Makeup Inspired by Winter: Winter makeup embraces richer, deeper tones that capture the magic of the season. To achieve a glowing complexion that contrasts well with the winter scenery, experiment with berry-toned lipsticks, smokey eyeshadows, and a hint of highlighter.

A celebration of the charm of the wintertime and the satisfaction of looking elegant while being warm. You may design outfits that capture the allure of winter and enable you to brave the chilly days with a sense of comfortable couture by embracing luxury layering, fun patterns, rich fabrics, and toasty accessories.

Part III: Dressing for Every Occasion

Chapter 7: Casual Guy: Elevating Your Everyday Attire

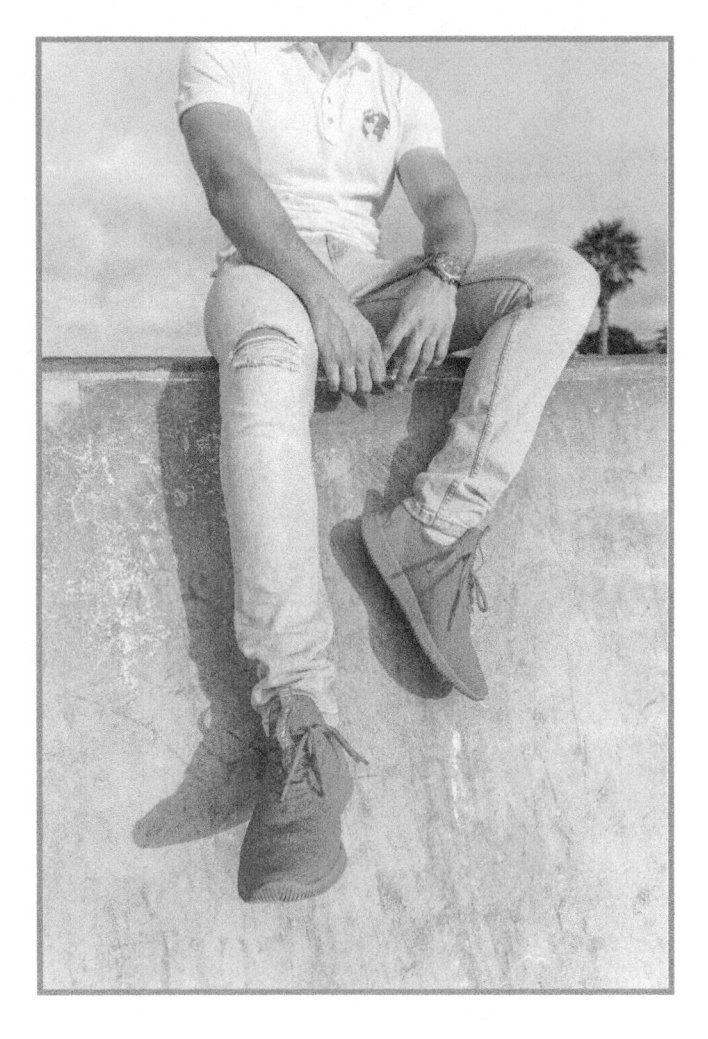

7.1 Effortless Cool: Navigating Casual Dress Codes

Casual clothing provides a platform for expressing your individual style while embracing a carefree attitude. The realm of casual dress rules calls for a careful balancing act between authenticity, comfort, and self-assurance. With tips on how to master the casual dress code while staying loyal to your individual style, this chapter digs into the art of seamlessly radiating coolness through your everyday attire.

The Power of Essentials: The foundation of casual dressing is assembling a wardrobe of adaptable essentials. Start with well-fitting chinos, casual shirts in muted colors, and jeans. These basic items act as a blank canvas on which to overlay and accessorize.

T-Shirts with a Twist: Choose premium materials and original patterns to up your T-shirt game. When worn with the appropriate bottoms and accessories, a well-fitted T-shirt may make a fashion statement. Look into graphic tees, textured materials, and subtle patterns to give your casual outfit more dimension.

Easy-going Footwear: Casual footwear needs to balance both comfort and fashion. Choose footwear that goes with your casual attire, such as spotless sneakers, desert boots, or loafers. These options give your regular appearance a little more refinement.

The Versatile Denim Jacket: A denim jacket adds a layer of elegance to your ensemble and is a casual necessity. For a lively and carefree look, combine it with T-shirts, button-down shirts, or even light sweaters.

Easy Layering: Casual attire benefits greatly from layering. Combine your essentials with breathable cardigans, hoodies, or even a sporty bomber jacket. Layering gives your clothing depth and aesthetic intrigue.

The Casual Way to Accessorize: You may add style to your casual clothing without sacrificing comfort. To inject some personality, choose a chic watch, a braided belt, or a straightforward bracelet. These minute nuances showcase your uniqueness while enjoying a relaxed atmosphere.

Easy Grooming: Easy grooming goes well with casual clothing. Depending on your desire, choose a clean shave or a well-kept beard to keep a well-groomed image. Keep your hair tidy and styled in a way that suits your laid-back appearance.

Summer Casual: Incorporate airy materials and eye-catching hues into your casual clothes to embrace the summer season. While keeping you cool and cozy, linen shirts, shorts, and espadrilles evoke the spirit of the season.

Winter Casual: Warm fabrics and layering are required for winter casual clothes. Choose insulating clothing like thermal henleys, flannel shirts, and chunky knit sweaters that are also stylish. To create a winter-ready style, pair these with tough boots or sneakers.

Athletic-Inspired Casual: The fusion of fashion and athleticism offers a distinctive approach to casual attire. To create a contemporary and exciting casual look, mix components from sportswear like joggers, performance sneakers, and sporty sweatshirts.

Embrace the trend of casual tailoring by fusing tailored clothing with more laid-back accessories. For an elegant yet laid-back appearance that goes from day to night, team a well-fitted blazer with dark trousers or chinos.

The ability to add effortless coolness to your everyday style can be found in casual clothes. You may design outfits that seamlessly encapsulate the spirit of casual elegance by mastering the art of essentials, experimenting with versatile footwear, embracing layering, and incorporating understated accessories. Whatever you're doing—running errands, visiting friends, or just taking the day off—your casual wardrobe reflects your unhurried confidence and unique style.

7.2 Dressing Down with Style: Beyond Denim and Tees

Even in the most laid-back environments, dressing down offers you the chance to show off your sartorial skill without losing style. This section delves into the art of dressing down with style, examining how to create looks that ooze charm and confidence using ordinary items like denim and T-shirts. You'll learn how to inject a dash of fashionable flair into your downtime, whether it be weekend adventures or casual outings.

Denim tact: The basis of wearing casually in style is denim. Try out several sizes, washes, and designs to create a collection of jeans that can be worn in a variety of situations. Denim provides a blank canvas for constructing adaptable outfits, from traditional straight-leg to slim-fit and distressed shapes.

The Perfect Tee: By emphasizing fit and materials, elevate the basic T-shirt. Select high-quality cotton t-shirts that fit you nicely and have a flattering drape. Simple patterns or solid colors can instantly upgrade your look.

Mastering the Casual Shirt: Beyond tees, casual shirts are essential for dressing down stylishly. Accept button-down shirts, henleys, and chambray shirts that combine comfort and style in the right amounts. These choices are adaptable enough to go with chinos or denim.

Dressing down requires understanding the technique of layering. Your outfit can be instantly improved by adding a light sweater, cardigan, or casual jacket while also adding depth and texture. When moving between indoor and outdoor situations, layering is extremely helpful.

The adaptable denim jacket: A mainstay in dressing down, the denim jacket is back. It goes great with a T-shirt, especially when layered with a hoodie or flannel shirt to give off a laid-back and friendly vibe.

Sneakers: Casual Essential Sneakers are the preferred footwear for casual attire. Choose timeless white sneakers, canvas shoes, or even simple leather shoes. You can wear them with a range of casual outfits because of their adaptability.

Chino Man: Chinos maintain a casual look while providing a polished alternative to denim. To create effortlessly fashionable outfits, go for slim-fit or straight-leg chinos in neutral colors. T-shirts, casual shirts, or thin sweaters are appropriate accompaniments.

sports Appeal: Incorporate sports apparel into your casual outfits to embrace sporty features. For an on-trend athletic-inspired outfit, track jackets, performance tees, and jogger trousers can be worn together smoothly.

Accentuating your wardrobe with accessories is important, even in informal settings. Choose a chic watch, a leather belt, or a straightforward bracelet to add some flair to your ensemble.

Easy Hairstyles: Dressing down requires similarly easy hairstyles. Accept natural hair texture, a tousled appearance, or a well-groomed appearance to go with your casual attire.

Weekend Getaway clothing: When organizing a weekend getaway, think of adaptable clothing that may be worn for a variety of activities. Choose clothing that is comfortable without sacrificing style for activities like exploring the city, hiking, or relaxing.

Your ability to adroitly combine comfort and style is demonstrated by your ability to dress down with flare. You can design outfits that effortlessly exude confidence and charm in every informal occasion by perfecting the art of denim, choosing the ideal tees and casual shirts, and experimenting with layering. Your downtime becomes an opportunity to express your distinctive design sensibility while feeling at ease in your wardrobe, whether it be coffee shop outings or leisurely strolls.

Chapter 8: The Art of Evening Glamour

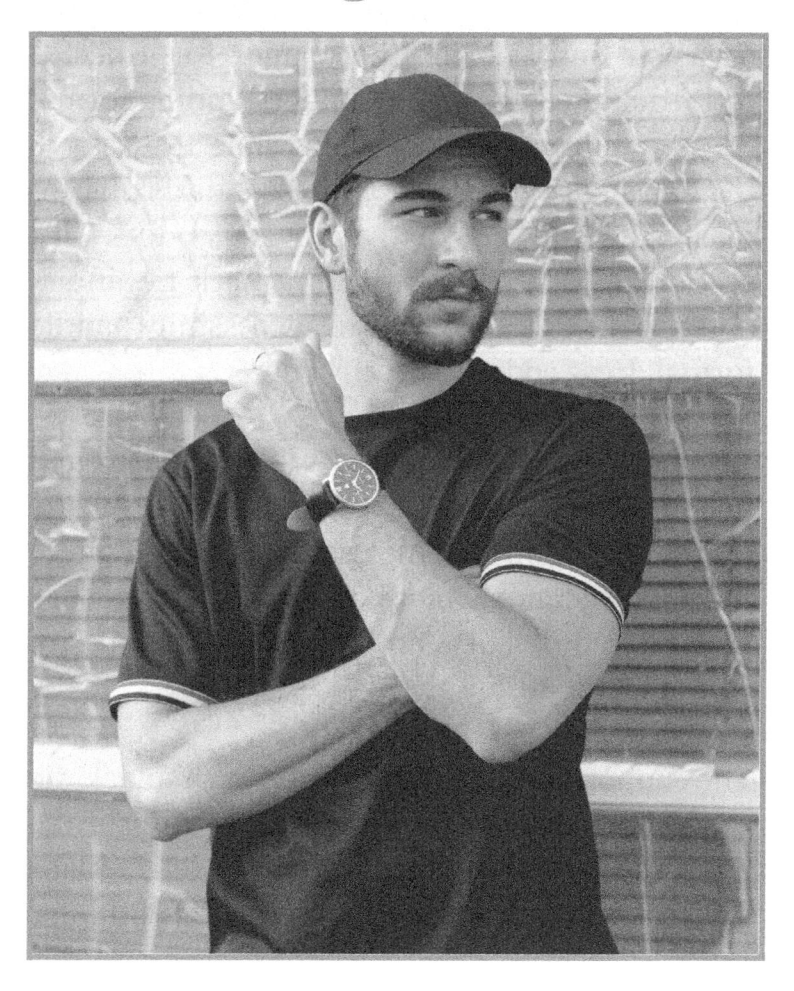

8.1 Black Tie Brilliance: Navigating Formal Dress Codes

Evening parties are seductive not only for the occasion but also for the chance to project a refined and elegant aura. Understanding formal dress requirements and being able to dress to the occasion's grandeur are essential skills for mastering the art of evening splendor. This section digs into the world of black tie affairs and provides tips on how to successfully handle formal dress codes.

The Elegance of Black Tie: A sophisticated and polished appearance is required for black tie occasions. Adopt a timeless black suit, a white dress shirt, and a black bow tie. This outfit's understated beauty and focus on detail are embodied in its simplicity.

The importance of accessories in a black tie ensemble can't be overstated. To finish the appearance, choose a formal dress watch, black patent leather shoes, and understated cufflinks.

These little additions enhance your look without taking away from the event's formality.

Dress Shirt Perfection: Within the constraints of formal wear, the dress shirt serves as a blank canvas for displaying your personal style. Select a white dress shirt with a spread or wing collar for an elegant touch. The attractiveness of your outfit is further enhanced by pleated front or French cuffs.

Adding Elevation with a Cummerbund: A cummerbund gives your black tie ensemble a touch of class. To complement your tuxedo perfectly, pick a cummerbund that is either black or a similar color. This accessory defines your waistline while also enhancing your outfit.

The Allure of a Waistcoat: Choose a waistcoat or vest to add depth to your outfit. A black or complementary waistcoat adds a traditional touch and a feeling of completion.

Grooming for Formality: For a black tie affair, you must look flawless. Make sure you look clean-shaven or well-groomed, and think about a sophisticated classic hairdo. Your dedication to the event is demonstrated by the care you take with your appearance.

Elegance and Confidence: Attending a black tie event successfully requires more than simply appropriate apparel. Along with your elegant appearance, radiate a sense of security by standing up straight, keeping a good posture, and standing tall.

8.2 Cocktail Connoisseur: Striking the Perfect Balance

Cocktail parties offer a distinctive venue for showcasing your personal style while finding the ideal harmony between formality and informal flare. Understanding the subtleties of the dress code and adding your own sense of flair to your wardrobe is key to mastering the art of cocktail wear. In this section, we examine how to create ensembles that perfectly encapsulate the event in order to become a cocktail connoisseur.

The Versatility of Cocktail Clothing: When compared to black tie events, cocktail clothing is more adaptable. Choose a suit in a dark hue like navy, charcoal, or deep gray that is well-fitted. Your cocktail outfit is built on a fitted two-piece suit.

Selecting a Shirt: Pick a dress shirt that matches your suit and is in a complementary hue. A variety of suit colors go nicely with classic choices like crisp white or light blue. For a modern touch, think about a spread or point collar.

Tie or No Tie: While a tie is typically worn with formal wear, there are other options available for cocktail occasions. Choose a silk or knit tie to add refinement to your outfit, or go tieless. The option you make will rely on the event's formality and your own preferences.

With the appropriate shoes, you can elevate your cocktail attire. Pick a pair of leather dress shoes or loafers that accentuate or match the color of your outfit. A balance between fashion and comfort should be achieved with the footwear.

Subtle Accessorizing: Accessorizing adds to the overall sophistication of your evening wear. Simple cufflinks, a dress watch, and a discreet pocket square give elegant accents without overpowering the look.

Excellence in grooming is required for cocktail occasions, and your appearance should match your clothing. Ensure a clean-shaven appearance, a nice haircut, and well-groomed facial hair. Your grooming routine should match the formality of the event.

Confidence and Charm: Cocktail attire is more than simply your appearance; it's how you carry yourself. Maintain a friendly grin, talk to people, and project approachability to enhance the social environment of the gathering.

Mastering the delicate balance between formal and casual elegance is a prerequisite for cocktail connoisseurship. You may design outfits that seamlessly capture the atmosphere of cocktail events by selecting a versatile suit, matching it with a well-fitted dress shirt, playing with tie alternatives, and accessorizing subtly. Your cocktail dress showcases your sharp fashion sense and improves your appearance at any social event, whether you're networking or celebrating a particular occasion.

Chapter 9: Groom and Groomsmen: The Perfect Wedding Ensemble

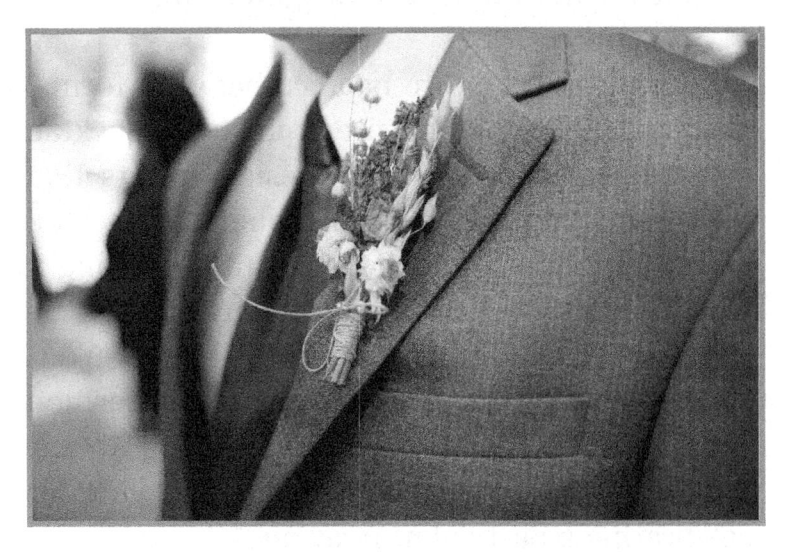

9.1 Dapper Grooming: Dressing for Your Big Day

Your wedding day is a significant event that necessitates dressing impeccably. As the groom, your attire should be a reflection of your unique taste and work with the celebration's overarching theme. This section digs into the finer points of dapper grooming and walks you through the steps of creating the ideal look for your wedding day that will make an impression.

The Ideal Suit: Opt for a suit that complements the wedding's formality and atmosphere. Choose traditional hues like black, navy, or charcoal, or for a daylight occasion, think of a lighter shade. Your physique should be highlighted by the suit's flawless fit.

Coordinating with the Theme: Your suit's color and style should go well with the wedding's theme, whether it's a formal ceremony or a rustic outdoor party. You can match your accessories, like ties, pocket squares, and boutonnieres, to the room's theme.

Choose a dress shirt that matches the color and design of the suit. Popular choices include bright white or a gentle pastel color. Make sure the shirt fits properly and complements the suit.

Whether to wear a tie or a bow tie depends on the level of formality of the occasion and your particular style. A bow tie provides a touch of sophistication while a traditional silk tie conveys timelessness in elegance.

Your choice of footwear should be both comfy and fashionable. Choose well-polished leather dress shoes that are the same color as the outfit. Before the big day, make sure the shoes are broken in.

Excellence in Grooming: Dressing for your wedding day requires more than simply grooming. To ensure a professional appearance, make an appointment for a haircut and grooming session a few days before the event. The style is finished off with perfectly manicured nails and a clean-shaven or well-groomed beard.

Poise and Confidence: Your appearance is just as vital as your manner. As you walk down the aisle, be sure to stand up straight, make eye contact, and project confidence and composure. The attractiveness of your outfit will be enhanced by your assurance.

9.2 The Groomsmen's Handbook: Coordinated Looks for a Memorable Event

A sign of your friendship and camaraderie is choosing a group of groomsmen who support your wedding style. By matching each other's outfits, you can create a stylish ensemble that improves the wedding's overall aesthetics. In order to make your wedding unique and well-matched, this section offers advice on selecting a coordinated style for your groomsmen.

Matching Color Scheme: Decide on a color scheme that goes with your groom's outfit as well as the wedding's overall theme. This color palette can be used by the groomsmen's outfits to create a uniform look.

Establish a dress code that is appropriate for the event's formality and stick to it. Make sure that all of the groomsmen wear attire that is at the same level of formality, whether that be suits, tuxedos, or something more casual.

Accessories that Promote Unity: The use of ties, bow ties, pocket squares, and boutonnieres can promote harmony among the groomsmen. By coordinating these components, you may create a unified appearance that goes well with the overall theme.

Pay Close Attention to Fit: Each groomsman's clothing should be sized specifically for their body type. A polished and sophisticated appearance is created by wearing clothing that fits properly.

guys Gifts: To show your appreciation for your guys, give them gifts or accessories that match their outfits. Personalized socks, tie bars, or cufflinks make excellent thank-you gifts.

Encourage the groomsmen to match their grooming habits to the level of formality of the occasion. Make appointments for haircuts, grooming sessions, and nail treatments to maintain a glossy and well-groomed image.

Teamwork and Unity: Stress the value of groomsmen working together as a team. Throughout the wedding day, promote friendly interactions, unity, and shared obligations.

Coordinating the groom and groomsmen's dress is an opportunity to demonstrate your attention to detail and produce a pleasing visual effect. You can build an ensemble that expresses your uniqueness and honors the joy you enjoyed on your wedding day with your groomsmen by choosing the ideal suit, coordinating with the wedding's theme, paying attention to grooming details, and encouraging unity among groomsmen. A memorable and elegant event will be remembered for years to come thanks to your dapper appearance and the groomsmen's synchronized style.

Chapter 10: Activewear Beyond the Gym: Athletic Excellence

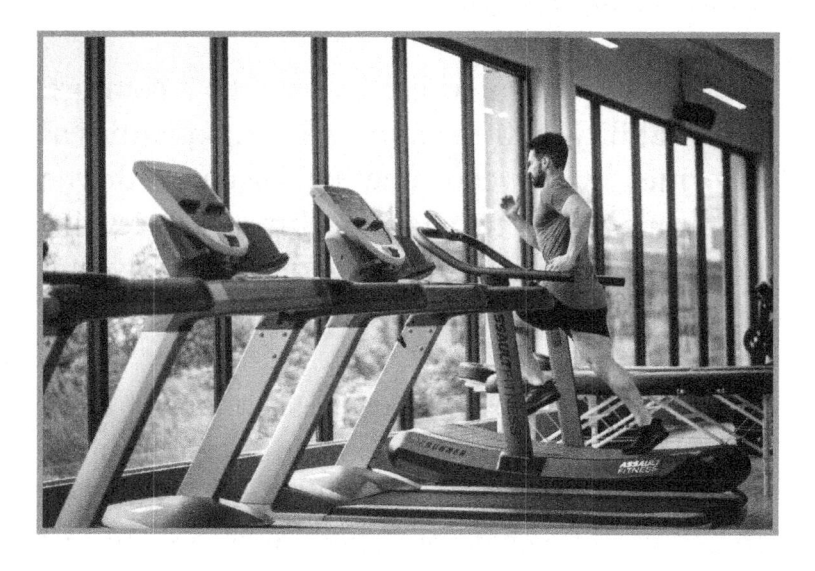

10.1 Sporty Fashion: Dressing for Comfort and Performance

Athletic greatness includes the ability to seamlessly incorporate sporty style into your daily wardrobe and goes beyond the boundaries of the gym or the playing field. Incorporating sports features into your clothing while putting performance, comfort, and a unique sense of style first is covered in this section. Achieving athletic style allows you to move with comfort and exude confidence throughout both active and relaxed outings.

Functional materials: Adopt comfort, breathability, and moisture-wicking qualities as priorities when choosing performance-driven materials. For active days, technical fabrics like moisture-wicking blends, nylon, and polyester offer the best functionality.

Performance Tops: Choose t-shirts, tank tops, or polo shirts that are designed for performance and allow for easy mobility and effective moisture management. These tees are perfect for both casual outings and workouts.

Active Bottoms: Joggers, track trousers, and athletic shorts are crucial elements of sports fashion. For functionality, look for bottoms with drawstrings, elastic waistbands, and functional pockets.

Layering for Versatility: Layering is important for creating an athletic appearance that works in a variety of circumstances. You may easily layer a thin zip-up jacket, a sweat-wicking sweatshirt, or a windbreaker over your activewear to add flair and functionality.

Sneakers are the cornerstone of sports fashion. They are footwear for action. Choose supportive, comfortable athletic shoes that are appropriate for your level of exercise. Your sneakers should offer both flair and functionality, whether you're running errands or playing a quick game of basketball.

Accessorizing the Active Look: Sporty apparel is complemented by minimal accessories. Consider adding a useful accessory to your look, such as a lightweight bag, a baseball cap, or a sporty watch.

10.2 Athleisure Aesthetics: Combining Sophistication with Sport

The art of fusing sporty aspects with sophisticated aesthetics to create an outfit that easily transitions from strenuous activities to social events is known as athleisure. This section delves into the specifics of athleisure and offers tips on how to create elegant yet sporty ensembles that command respect.

Tracksuits have advanced to become fashionable athleisure essentials. Select tracksuits with subtle patterns or monochromatic coloring and precise cuts that convey class. For a stylish and put-together look, team them with a spotless pair of sneakers.

Joggers have evolved from being gym attire to a multipurpose athleisure item. Choose well-fitting joggers made of luxurious materials that flow gracefully. For a stylish yet laid-back appearance, wear them with a loose button-down shirt or a thin sweater.

Polo shirts with a performance focus: Polo shirts with a performance focus blend sportiness with classic elegance. Pick polo shirts made of technology fabrics for moisture control and a refined appearance.

Combining Sport Coats: Formal and athletic clothing can even be worn together. Try wearing a fitted blazer or sport coat with joggers or pants with an athletic vibe. This unanticipated blending of athletics and luxury results in a unique and stylish combination.

Monochromatic Magic: To enhance the sophistication of your athleisure appearance, embrace a monochromatic color scheme. Cohesive color schemes produce an aesthetic that is pleasing to the eye.

Functional Accessories: To complete the casual-yet-sophisticated vibe of your outfit, accessorize with a leather belt, a sleek pair of sunglasses, or a minimalist timepiece.

Athleisure aesthetics should be embraced while exuding grace and confidence. Stand tall, project confidence, and converse with others in a laid-back manner.

Mastering athletic excellence through activewear involves more than just wearing clothes; it is adopting a way of life that puts comfort, performance, and style first. You may create an athleisure aesthetic, choose functional materials, embrace sports tops and bottoms, layer wisely, and create a versatile wardrobe that seamlessly goes from casual outings to active pursuits. Your sports aesthetic becomes a reflection of your vivacious personality and aptitude for fusing style and utility.

Part IV: Crafting Confidence Through Style

Chapter 11: The Confidence Code: Dressing for Self-Assurance

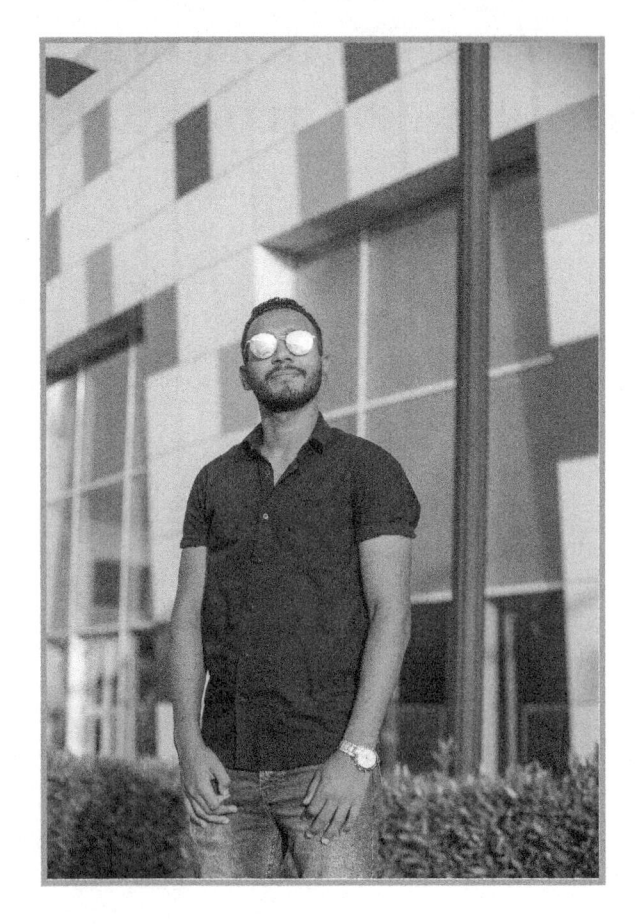

11.1 Unlocking Self-Esteem Through Your Wardrobe

Dressing is a powerful instrument that can have a beneficial effect on your internal state and is not just an exterior act. The profound relationship between clothing choices and self-esteem is explored in this section. You can access a reservoir of confidence that radiates from within by purposefully choosing clothing that connects with your true self and flatters your body type.

Authentic Expression: You can use your clothes as a canvas to show the world who you are and what you stand for. You can project authenticity by dressing in a way that speaks to your personality, hobbies, and objectives.

Clothing that flatters your body type and highlights your best features should be worn. Dressing to accentuate your physique boosts your self-esteem, whether it's via understanding your proportions or selecting well-fitted clothing.

Dressing Up Your Mood Colors and textiles have a big influence on how you feel. Try out various shades and textures to conjure feelings of assurance, optimism, and self-assurance.

Create a collection of clothes that you connect with inspiring moments or satisfying memories to start building your self-esteem wardrobe. Wearing these goods boosts your self-confidence and gives you a sense of success.

11.2 How to Dress Confidently in Today's World

A wardrobe that exudes self-assurance and versatility is necessary for navigating the challenges of the modern world. This part looks at how to put together groups that give you the confidence and charm to handle social and professional situations.

Create a professional wardrobe that radiates expertise and power by dressing with confidence. Accept crafted suits, clean dress shirts, and polished shoes that demonstrate your dedication to quality.

Adapting to Modern Trends: Keeping up with modern fashion trends enables you to combine relevance and flair. Keep your distinct style while incorporating modern components into your clothing.

Dress appropriately for the occasion: Knowing what to wear for different settings gives you the power to leave a lasting impression. When you dress appropriately, whether, for a business meeting, social event, or casual trip, your confidence will increase.

Creating a Signature Look: Having a distinctive look makes getting ready easier while improving your feeling of self. Determine the essential components and features that resonate with you and become associated with your personal brand.

Chapter 12: Fit and Fabulous: Dressing for Different Body Types

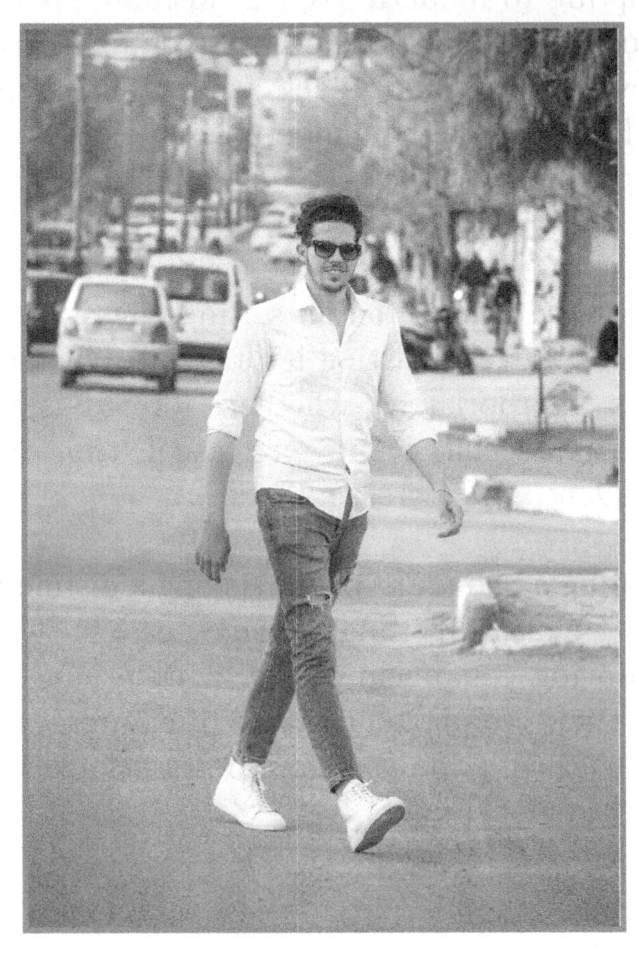

12.1 Finding Your Perfect Fit: Celebrating Diversity

The pursuit of style is an opportunity to embrace your originality and enjoy the distinctive features of your body. This section looks into the art of dressing for various body types, including tips and tricks to highlight your assets, reduce weaknesses, and put together an outfit that boosts your self-assurance and appeal.

Recognize your body type, whether it is ectomorph, mesomorph, or endomorph, and become familiar with its traits. You can choose apparel that flatters your proportions with this knowledge.

Ectomorphs should choose apparel that adds visual weight and volume if their form is slim and angular. The appearance of a bigger body is simulated via layering, structured jackets, and textured materials.

Mesomorphs should embrace their balanced and athletic build with well-fitting clothing that draws attention to their proportions. The natural symmetry of your body is highlighted with tailored clothing such as suits, shirts, and tapered pants.

Selecting clothing for endomorphs includes finding balance and definition while dressing for a softer and rounded profile. Darker hues, vertical patterns, and structural pieces enhance your style while having a slimming effect.

Highlighting Your Assets: Take note of your physical strengths and wear attire that emphasizes them. Strategic clothing choices highlight your best features, whether they are broad shoulders, a defined waist, or strong legs.

Challenges that require concealment: Subtly address any areas you would want to reduce. Choose clothes shapes and styles that deflect attention away from these regions while still creating a cohesive look.

Play with proportions by being aware of the ideas of balance and proportion when choosing your clothing. A unified and visually appealing design is produced by using elements like contrasting colors, layering, and clever accessories.

Triumph of Tailoring: To ensure that your clothes fit perfectly, invest in professional tailoring. Whatever your body shape, tailored clothing enhances your silhouette and gives you a sophisticated look.

Experimenting with Style: Adopt trends that work for your body shape and embrace experimentation. Make sure you seem current and flattering by adapting current fashion trends to your unique style.

You may unlock the power of dressing to improve your individual qualities by embracing the variety of body shapes and learning how to choose clothes that flatter your figure. Dressing for your body type is about more than just looking good; it's also about accepting your uniqueness and fostering a greater feeling of self-acceptance.

12.2 Tailoring Advice: How to Dress for Your Individual Body

The secret weapon that turns ordinary clothing into extraordinary combinations that accentuate your body's proportions and characteristics is tailoring. This section digs into the subject of tailoring and offers helpful tips and methods to optimize the fit of your wardrobe and make sure that each piece of clothing complements your unique body type and sense of style.

Professional alterations: Develop a relationship with a talented tailor who can effectively analyze the subtleties of your body and change items for a perfect fit. Professional modifications improve your appearance regardless of whether they are made into shirts, coats, or pants.

Customization for Elegance: If you want the highest level of customization, consider purchasing made-to-measure or bespoke clothing. These specialized garments are made for your body, ensuring a perfect fit and a sophisticated silhouette.

The art of the jacket and blazer: Well-tailored jackets and blazers lay gently on your shoulders and drape beautifully. Your physique will be enhanced and you'll look more sleek with the right sleeve length and waist suppression.

Perfect pants: A well-groomed outfit must include tailored trousers. Get the optimum waist fit, leg breadth, and pant length to highlight your lower body while preserving freedom of movement.

Success with the Shirt: By removing extra fabric and guaranteeing a crisp silhouette, tailored shirts give off a polished impression. Your upper body is complemented with a well-fitting shirt, which improves your posture and self-assurance.

Suit Sophistication: A suit can be tailored to become a sartorial masterpiece from just an ordinary outfit. To produce a unified and aesthetically pleasing look, the suit's shoulders, sleeves, jacket length, and trouser fit are all precisely modified.

Precision Layering: The cornerstone for layering is tailored components. Layered outfits are given structure by jackets, blazers, and vests while still looking classy and put together.

Accentuating with accessories: Tailoring includes accessories. Make an investment in belts, ties, and pocket squares that balance out the proportions of your ensemble.

Confident Carriage: Your body language should reflect the enhanced impression that a fitted outfit exudes. To show off the perfectly cut details of your clothing, stand tall, keep a straight stance, and move easily.

By utilizing tailoring tactics and ideas, you may maximize the fit and appreciate the uniqueness of the body form of your clothing. Clothing is transformed via the technique of tailoring into a unique expression of style that enhances your proportions and emanates self-assurance. Enhance your image by wearing tailored clothes that not only suit your body type but also demonstrate your attention to detail and dedication to dressing elegantly.

Chapter 13: The Power of Accessories: Upgrading Every Look

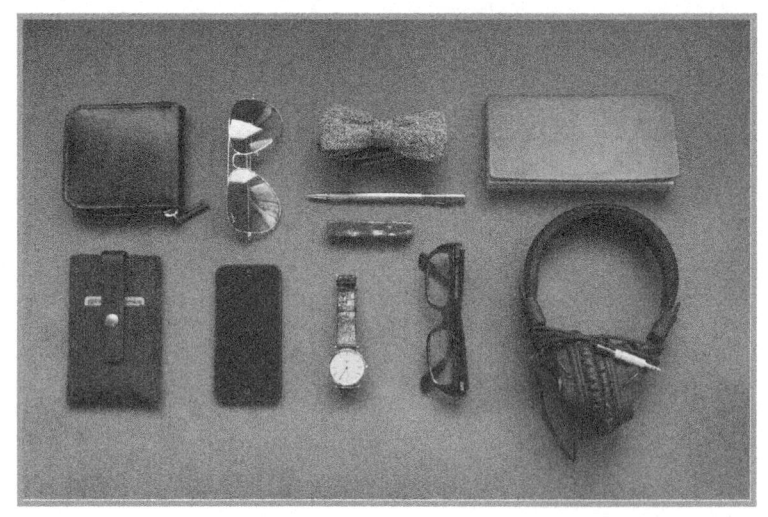

Accessories have the amazing power to elevate a simple outfit into a unique expression of individuality and style. The art of accessorizing is explored in depth in this chapter, along with the numerous ways that well-chosen accessories can define and elevate your appearance, giving you the chance to leave a lasting impression and project confidence at all times.

13.1 Getting the Hang of Men's Accessories: Watches and Wallets

The Wristwatch Wonder: A wristwatch goes beyond being merely functional to become a representation of style and sophistication. The proper watch acts as an extension of your personality and taste, whether it's a traditional dress watch, a functional chronograph, or a striking statement piece.

Bracelet Brilliance: Wristbands and bracelets give you the chance to add character and texture to your outfit. These small modifications, like metal bands or leather cuffs, improve the aesthetic attractiveness of your wrist and support your personal fashion statement.

Neckwear Details Neckties, bow ties, and neckerchiefs add character and panache to your outfit. Select patterns, materials, and knot techniques that complement the concept of your ensemble and exude refinement.

Belts are being redefined: Belts are no longer just useful accessories; they have evolved into embellishments that complete your look. To create a unified and eye-catching style, experiment with various materials, textures, and buckle designs.

Wallet Advice: A well-made wallet conveys your attention to detail and organizational skills. Choose high-quality leather wallets that show craftsmanship, durability, and a hint of elegance.

13.2 The Magic of Ties, Pocket Squares, and More: The Subtle Impact

Neckties are more than just fashion items; they are means of communication. Make use of patterns, colors, and fabrics to match the setting and enhance your clothing. Learning several knot styles gives your appearance more flair and sophistication.

Poetry on Pocket Squares: Your jacket's breast pocket comes to life with artistic embellishments on pocket squares. Try different folds, patterns, and fabrics to give your outfit more style and personality.

Cufflinks and Studs: Cufflinks and studs that elevate your dress shirt and suit are appropriate for formal occasions. Choose patterns that reflect your individual taste, whether it is timeless elegance or cutting-edge modernism.

Tie bars and collar pins: These understated accessories have both practical and fashionable uses. A collar pin raises the collar of your dress shirt and adds a touch of classic elegance, while a tie bar keeps your tie in place and adds polish.

Sock Sensations: Socks offer a platform for exhibiting character and originality. It's possible to make a statement in even the smallest details when using striking hues, fun patterns, and intriguing textures.

Accessories as Conversation Starters: Carefully selected accessories present chances for lively discussions. Items that are one-of-a-kind, vintage treasures, or have sentimental worth can serve as conversation starters by showcasing your hobbies and passions.

The Balancing Act: Although accessories improve your appearance, moderation is important. Achieve a well-balanced accessory collection that enhances your look without overpowering it.

Wearing carefully chosen accessories not only improves your appearance but also makes you feel more confident. Knowing that you've

138

painstakingly chosen your wardrobe with attention to detail gives you the confidence to handle social situations with ease.

Curating a collection of accessories that complement your particular style and heighten the effect of your outfit is the key to mastering the art of accessorizing. Wristwatches, bracelets, neckpieces, belts, wallets, and other accessories are expertly incorporated into your outfits to elevate them above the ordinary and produce a visual story that expresses your style and personality in great detail. With the help of accessories, you can confidently express yourself, draw attention to yourself, and make an impression that will endure long after you leave the place.

Chapter 14: Fragrance and Beyond A Scent of Distinction

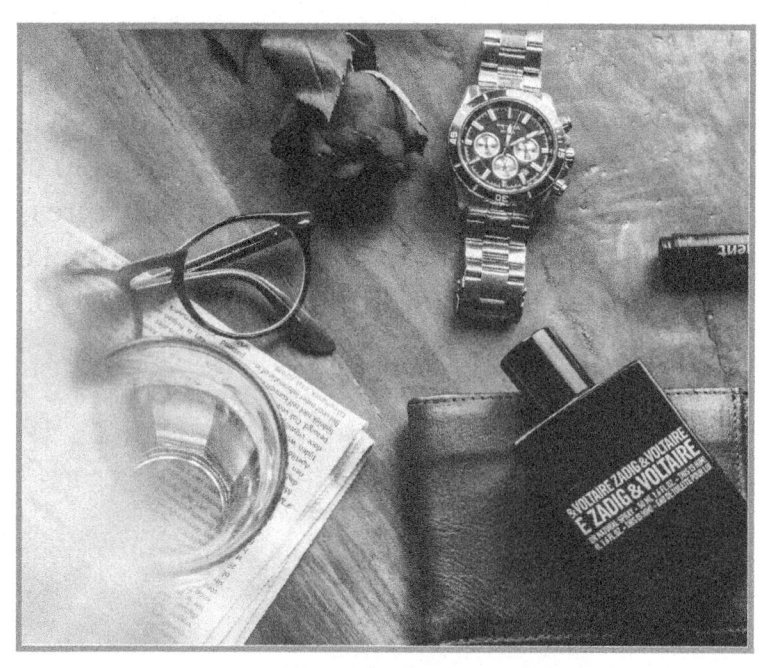

Fragrance, sometimes known as the "invisible accessory," has the unmatched power to arouse feelings, bring back memories, and leave an everlasting impression. This chapter goes deeply into the alluring world of fragrances, examining men's grooming basics, the art of men's fragrance, and the significant effects that a well-chosen perfume can have on your overall appearance and self-assurance.

14.1 Men's Fragrance: The Art of a Signature Scent

Scent Identity: Your preferred fragrance helps to identify your individual olfactory identity, just as your personal style of clothes does. An extension of your personality, a signature perfume resonates with who you are and leaves a magical trail wherever you go.

Understanding the various fragrance families, such as citrus, woody, oriental, aquatic, and more, gives you the power to choose smells that go with various events and seasons, boosting your presence with a pleasing perfume.

The Symphony of the Notes: Top, middle, and base notes all play a part in the development of a fragrance. Accept odors that evolve over time, mesmerizing others with a complex olfactory experience.

Developing a Signature perfume: The search for a signature perfume entails exploration and experimenting. Choose a scent that truly resonates with you and inspires favorable responses from people around you after trying a variety of them and allowing them to interact with your skin chemistry.

Techniques for Application: Strategically applying scent increases its impact. Pay attention to the wrists, neck, and area behind the ears as these are pulse points that release heat and intensify scents to create a constant and alluring atmosphere.

Practice fragrance etiquette by applying your fragrance discreetly. Your aroma should complement the surroundings rather than dominate them. A thoughtfully chosen scent leaves a lasting impression, creating a favorable connection to your presence.

14.2 Deodorants, colognes, and Grooming Routines: The Essentials

Effective underarm care is the cornerstone of your fragrance journey, according to underarm elegance. Choose deodorants that work well with your selected cologne and offer all-day freshness and odor protection.

Choosing the Right Cologne: Spend money on colognes that fit your personality and sense of style. A timeless elegance can be found in classic colognes, while a new allure can be found in scents.

Layering to Extend Life: Use grooming items that go well with your selected cologne to extend its life and impact. A consistent and long-lasting olfactory experience can be produced by matching shower gels, body lotions, and deodorants.

Daily Grooming Rituals: Create a grooming schedule that fits your way of life. A well-groomed canvas for your preferred fragrance is created by frequent bathing, moisturizing, and beard maintenance.

Fragrance is a subtle, personal expression that is meant to be detected by those who are nearby. Choose discretion when applying, letting them catch alluring hints of you as you move.

Grooming as Self-Care: Grooming goes beyond the surface; it is a self-respecting activity. Your confidence is boosted by having a well-groomed appearance, which enables you to handle difficulties with grace and poise.

By mastering the art of men's fragrances and embracing grooming necessities, you may boost your presence and appearance by utilizing the transformational power of scents. Those who come into contact with you will always remember you because of the scent you've chosen. A signature aroma and rigorous grooming practices work together to produce a full sensory experience that boosts your self-confidence, improves your appearance, and leaves a trace of elegance and charm wherever you go.

14.3 Choosing and Using Body Sprays, Deodorants, and Fragrances for Various Situations

The scent is a crucial yet frequently disregarded aspect of your entire appearance. The ideal scent may make an impression and improve your presence. The skill of choosing and utilizing body sprays, deodorants, and perfumes to enhance your style and confidence is covered in this section.

Choosing the Right Fragrance: You should be very selective here, Pick a scent that fits your personality and or the occasion's mood. To make wise decisions, become familiar with fragrance families.

Scents and Occasions: Scents should be chosen according to the occasion. Choose lighter, more airy perfumes for daytime activities, saving the stronger, more intoxicating scents for evening occasions.

Layering for Longevity: Layer your fragrance with scented care items like deodorants and body sprays to extend its potency. This improves the overall impact and makes sure the smell profile is constant.

Apply perfumes sparingly, concentrating on pulse spots like the neck, the back of the ears, and the wrists. A nice and understated presence is ensured by a subdued and evenly applied application.

You can maximize the potential of dressing as a self-assurance tool by developing self-esteem through your wardrobe, mastering confidence in the contemporary world, and grasping the subtleties of fragrance selection and application. You may navigate the obstacles of life with a renewed feeling of purpose and confidence when your clothing selections reflect your inner strength and sincerity.

Chapter 15:
Trendspotting: Including Contemporary Fashion in Your Wardrobe

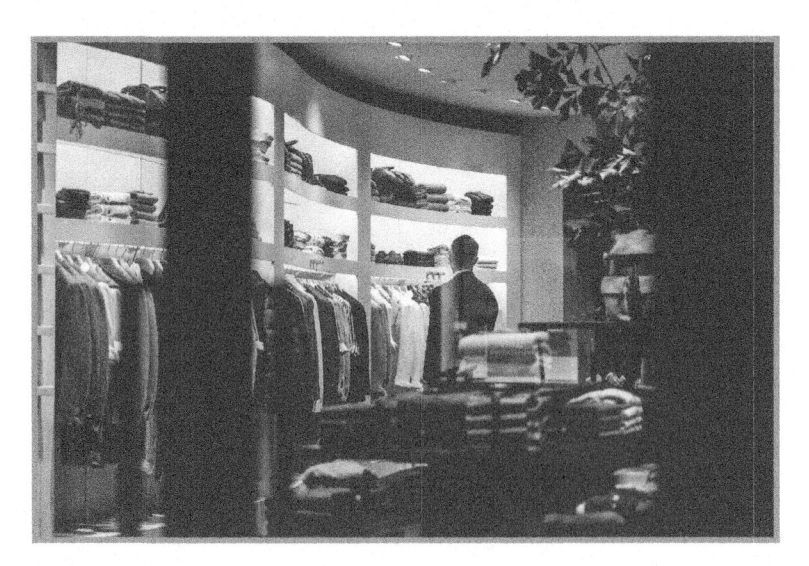

15.1 Interpreting Runway Trends: Adding High Fashion to Everyday Outfits

Fashion is a dynamic and always-changing industry that offers a never-ending stream of trends that both challenge and inspire. In order to stay current and express your originality through your clothing choices, this chapter discusses the art of trendspotting and the deft integration of high fashion concepts into your everyday wardrobe.

Understanding Trends: From cuts and colors to materials and patterns, trends are born on the catwalks of the world's fashion capitals. You can make decisions that fit your particular style by being aware of the cyclical nature of trends.

Adapting to Your Aesthetic: Although runway trends may appear avant-garde, the key is to make them fit your personal style. Find trends that fit with your personal style narrative and reinterpret them in a way that seems natural and harmonious.

Accessorizing: Accessorizing offers a method to experiment with trends without committing to a complete outfit change. To give your outfit a contemporary edge, incorporate trendy accessories like bold belts, futuristic eyewear, or unusual headgear.

Color Chronicles: In trend cycles, colors are crucial. You can add a contemporary touch to formal attire by experimenting with color schemes influenced by current trends in ties, pocket squares, and even shoes.

Print Expertise: Vibrant designs and patterns typically adorn catwalks. To get a dramatic yet well-balanced look, include trend-inspired prints sparingly, such as a printed shirt under a classic jacket or patterned socks with tailored pants.

Fabric Fantasia: Accent pieces or accessories are a subtle way to integrate trendy fabrics like metallics, velvets, or avant-garde textiles. These materials give your ensemble a mysterious and avant-garde flair.

Casual Elegance: Incorporating trendy components into casual ensembles is one approach to translating runway trends into everyday wear. An eclectic yet chic style can be created by mixing athletic clothing with traditional accessories like distressed jeans with a tailored blazer.

Innovative Layering: Adding layers to your outfits is a flexible method to incorporate runway trends. Try out different layering arrangements to give your current items fresh life.

Footwear Flourish: Shoes are a blank canvas on which to experiment with fashion. Your shoe choices can mirror the newest runway trends while enhancing your entire style, from clunky sneakers to unusual loafers.

Timeless with a Twist: Finding the right mix between modernism and timelessness is key to incorporating runway trends into your wardrobe. A well-fitted suit and a trendy tie, or a timeless white shirt and a modern pocket square, both show mastery of this mix.

Building Confidence: It takes self-assurance and confidence to adopt trends that are influenced by the runway. A trend that is successfully incorporated emanates modern elegance and makes a statement that is exclusively yours.

By understanding runway trends and incorporating high fashion ideas into your everyday attire, you may use your wardrobe as a blank canvas for your artistic expression. By keeping up with current trends and experimenting with novel aesthetics, you may maintain your sense of personal style. You can traverse the always-changing world of fashion with ease if you learn how to incorporate modern fashion into your wardrobe. You'll also be able to make sure that your sartorial selections reflect your personality, confidence, and openness to accept innovation.

15.2 Vintage Vibes: Reviving Timeless Pieces in Contemporary Ways

Fashion has a cyclical character, with older trends reviving and enthralling contemporary audiences. In this part, we look at how to incorporate vintage-inspired elements into your modern wardrobe to give classic pieces new life while yet retaining a current and fashionable look.

Rediscovering Timeless Elegance: Antiques have an unmatched sense of craftsmanship and history. Look for classic pieces that may be worn today and in the past, such as leather jackets, trench coats, and tailored suits.

Modern Interpretation: This is the secret to incorporating old things into your outfit. To put together a balanced and appealing look, pair a vintage jacket with modern slim-fit trousers or complement a timeless shirt with a current tie.

Adding old components with Accessories: Accessories offer the perfect backdrop for adding old components. In addition to paying respect to the past, wearing a pocket watch, suspenders, or a traditional leather briefcase will also give your appearance a unique charm.

Mixing periods: Play around with a fusion of periods by putting contemporary items next to vintage ones. For a fascinating fusion of styles, team up a vintage leather jacket with a modern turtleneck or a traditional fedora with modern streetwear.

Denim Dynamics: Denim, a classic material, works well for ensembles with a retro feel. For a casually stylish and classic look, add old denim jackets, pants, or vests to your outfit.

The perfect pattern can be blended into modern styles, such as houndstooth, herringbone, or pinstripes. To make a statement, wear a vintage-inspired jacket with plain pants or a contemporary tie.

Vintage-inspired shoes, like brogues, wingtips, or Chelsea boots, convey a timeless elegance that pairs well with contemporary outfits. These adaptable pieces fit numerous looks perfectly.

Textural Triumphs: Traditional features can be contrasted visually and tactilely with vintage materials like tweed, corduroy, and wool. For an air of refinement, add old textures with blazers, vests, or overcoats.

Vintage color schemes induce feelings of nostalgia, according to Color Chronicles Revisited. To create a harmonic interplay of shades, fill your wardrobe with vintage-inspired hues like earthy tones, soft pastels, or deep jewel tones.

Confident blending: The secret to vintage-inspired clothing's allure is in the eras' seamless blending. Infuse your ensemble with a modern sensibility while honoring the rich history of classic items to create a look that is both timeless and current.

A Timeless Statement: Adding vintage elements to your outfit demonstrates your respect for fashion history and your ability to give classic pieces new life. Your distinctive fusion of traditional and contemporary features reflects your refined taste and innovative attitude.

You honor the tradition of fashion while establishing your own style narrative by updating classic pieces in modern ways. The ability to create ensembles that express your identity, pay homage to the past, and garner appreciation in the present is made possible by the art of fusing old aesthetics with modern sensibilities, which transcends fashion fads.

Chapter 16: Style Evolution: Adapting to Changing Trends

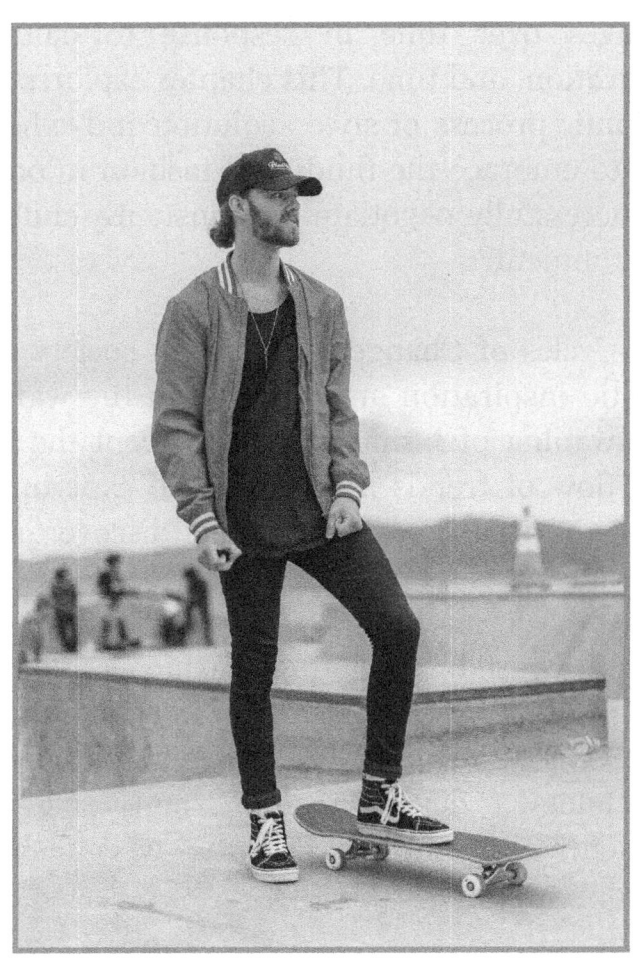

16.1 Adopting Fashion's Fluidity: Dressing for the Future

Fashion is a dynamic, living creature that changes over time in response to culture, innovation, and time. This chapter explores the dynamic process of style evolution and exhorts you to embrace the fluidity of fashion in order to successfully negotiate the constantly shifting environment.

The Cycles of Change: Changes in society and artistic inspiration are reflected in the waxing and waning of fashion trends. Accept the ebb and flow of trends as a chance to experiment with your particular style and discover new aesthetics.

Future-focused: Adopting fashion's fluidity implies looking to the future while valuing the past. Keep an eye out for new designers, technology developments, and cultural influences that will affect the next fashion trend.

Reimagining the Classics: The foundation for adjusting to shifting trends is provided by classic pieces. Reimagine conventional components with contemporary interpretations to keep your design ageless while embracing new components.

Cultural Exchange: Globalization has democratized the fashion industry and allowed a fusion of various influences. Take inspiration from other cultures, embrace cross-cultural aesthetics, and fill your wardrobe with a rich tapestry of international fashions.

Sustainable Fashion: As the industry develops, so does our understanding of how it affects the environment. Support ethical brands, choose quality over quantity, and engage in the circular fashion industry to embrace sustainable methods.

16.2 A Journey of Style Adaptation: Balancing Trends and Timelessness

The Harmony of Hybrid: A harmonious fusion is necessary to strike a balance between fashion and timeless design. To create an outfit that emanates contemporary while maintaining timeless charm, pair a trend-driven piece with basic staples.

Approach trends as an experiment in self-expression when observing them. Make sure a trend complements rather than overpowers your entire appearance by incorporating it into your wardrobe and evaluating its resonance with your style narrative.

Create a collection of enduring distinctive essentials by following this advice. A well-fitted suit, a functional topcoat, or a classic watch are timeless elements that act as an anchor while letting you embrace passing fashions with ease.

Accessorizing with Trends: Accessorizing with trends offers a low-risk platform. To add a touch of modernity to your outfit, experiment with trend-inspired accessories like striped socks, distinctive ties, or eye-catching cufflinks.

Triumph of Tailoring: Tailoring is a potent tool for striking a balance between timelessness and trends. The lifespan of fashion-forward pieces is increased by a customized fit, which also ensures that they flow naturally into your entire style.

Cross-cultural fashion fusion is evidence of the adaptability of fashion. Accept clothing from all ethnic origins, appreciate and respect it for what it is, and incorporate it into your wardrobe.

Evolutionary Confidence: The process of style adaptation is evidence of your growing self-assurance and readiness to venture into uncharted waters. Keeping up with emerging trends demonstrates your adaptable nature and capacity for expansion.

You traverse the road of style growth with subtlety and grace by accepting the flexibility of fashion and striking a balance between trends and classics. Your capacity to adapt becomes a reflection of your commitment to respect tradition while embracing innovation, and your changing clothing tells a tale of creative experimentation and personal development. Your ability to blend the old with the modern becomes a defining characteristic of your timeless style as you confidently advance into the future.

Conclusion: Embrace Your Dapper Destiny

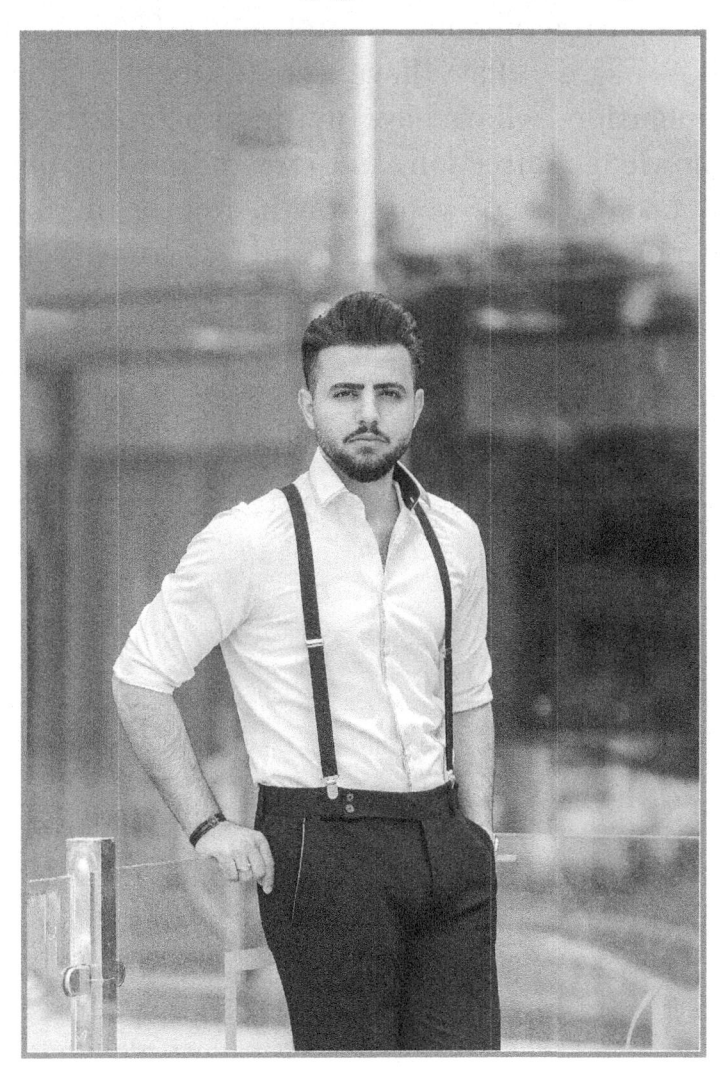

You stand at the beginning of a new chapter in your style adventure as we bring this sartorial odyssey to a close. You have been guided through the complex web of men's fashion on the pages that have come before this conclusion, which have unfurled a tapestry of knowledge, direction, and inspiration. It's time to take stock of your growth, rejoice in your increased self-assurance, and welcome your handsome future.

Enhance Your Everyday with Elegance: A Reminder to Keep Traveling in Style

You can paint your stories, your objectives, and your indomitable spirit onto any carefully chosen outfit. You convey a sense of assurance, composure, and appreciation for the creativity that goes into every stitch and fabric selection by donning the armor of style. The transformational effect that your clothing has on your manner, interactions, and sense of self-worth are what gives style its power, not just the clothes themselves.

A Life of Endless Exploration: Learning how to wear men's fashion well is like starting a lifelong adventure of exploration. You learn more about yourself with each stage, deepening your comprehension of what connects with your own identity. Continue to look for inspiration from people or things that ignite your enthusiasm, whether they be modern trendsetters, historical fashion heroes, or cultural aesthetics that speak to your soul.

A Versatile Wardrobe: Your wardrobe is a living representation of your development. Your style adapts and prospers as the seasons change and fashion trends shift. It is a collection of memories, encounters, and decisions that showcase your uniqueness. The varied persona that is distinctively yours can be captured by cultivating a wardrobe that adapts to occasions, climates, and trends with ease.

The legacy of confidence: The ultimate adornment, confidence is a silent but obvious declaration of self-assurance. With the information you've learned from these pages, you are now equipped with the skills necessary to conduct yourself confidently whether you're interacting with people in boardrooms, social settings, or casual settings. Your excellent look serves as a symbol of your inner fortitude and the unwavering confidence that radiates from you.

Walking the Dapper route: The route you've chosen is one that requires constant improvement. Recognize that even the most seasoned sartorialists are continual students of the craft, and accept your fresh style with humility and grace. Through the use of clothing, you have the freedom to experiment, develop, and express your uniqueness every day.

Making a Statement: You have definitely seen how men's fashion has evolved from a static means of self-expression to a dynamic means of wardrobe choice as you have traveled through these chapters. It's time to create your own chapter in the history of men's fashion now that you have the resources to put together your own unique look. Every flawlessly fitted suit, every carefully chosen accessory, and every tastefully put-together outfit becomes your mark of distinction and a declaration of your dedication to embracing your handsome destiny.

I welcome you to share your experience if this book has served as your mentor if its ideas have struck a chord with you, and if its observations have improved your understanding of men's fashion. Giving a favorable review is a way to share the knowledge and empowerment you've acquired, as well as to express your gratitude.

Another gentleman might be motivated by your review to start his own sartorial metamorphosis, giving him the chance to enjoy the assurance, charm, and refinement that come with accepting his handsome destiny.

Remember that style is a lifelong experience rather than a destination once the last page flips. Every day presents an opportunity to create a brand-new work of art on the canvas that is your wardrobe. Your fashion journey is a symphony of fabric and form, a tribute to the classic elegance you embody. Go forth, my reader, and confidently embrace your stylish destiny because your personal style is a lasting monument to your character and the legacy you leave behind.

Epilogue: Your Personal Style Manifesto

Style arises as a thread that connects your personality, aspirations, and confidence in the vast fabric of life. It's time to reaffirm your dedication to a personal style that captures your identity and welcomes the dynamic transformation that lies ahead as you stand at the conclusion of this enlightening journey.

Create your own style statement and accept that fashion is constantly evolving.

Making your own personal style statement is similar to writing a manifesto that expresses your uniqueness. In a world teeming with visual narratives, your declaration—etched through each clothing selection—becomes your signature. It's a tribute to the person you've grown to be, a proclamation of the course you intend to take, and an ode to the principles you uphold.

The Essence of Confidence: Personal style is more than just outward appearances; it's an expression of confidence that shines through in all of your actions and eye contact. Your clothing selections serve as a self-assurance shield as you enter each day, enabling you to face problems with a confident heart and a head held high.

An ode to authenticity: Your style is a reflection of your true self, a way that you convey your authenticity. Each shoe, tie, and piece of jewelry adds a different brushstroke to the portrait of your character. It's evidence that you take pride in all of your personality traits, weaknesses, and strengths.

Evolving Elegance: Your style manifesto is a threshold to the infinite possibilities of fashion, not a finish. Accept the continual growth with open arms because since fashion is constantly evolving, so should your personal style. Accept new fashion trends, try out creative outfit combinations, and inject some adventure into your wardrobe.

The Absolute Truth Perhaps a nagging query sprang to mind as you browse these pages: "Can every man truly dress great?" Without a doubt, every man has the ability to radiate brilliance through his appearance. Every guy can go on a journey of style change, just as you have traversed these chapters, honing your understanding and developing your taste.

Imagine a world in which each guy walked with purpose, radiating confidence, and embracing his individual flair. Your dedication to mastering men's fashion will have an impact on everyone around you in addition to being a personal journey for you. Your grace leaves a lasting impression, influencing future generations and inspiring others to use fashion as a means of self-expression and confidence.

Remember that your style manifesto—a harmonic fusion of the past, present, and future—is a living monument to your progress when you conclude this book. As a symbol of your identity, your hobbies, and your objectives, embrace it, celebrate it, and bring it with you wherever you go. May your individual sense of style serve as a tribute to your uniqueness, a record of your life's experiences, and a reminder that everyone can look fantastic in a suit and that includes them.

Made in United States
Orlando, FL
19 July 2024